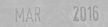

FOR THE LOVE OF FOOD AND YOGA

Skyhorse Publishing books may be purchased in bulk at special discounts for sales promotion, corporate gifts, fund-raising, or educational purposes. Special editions can also be created to specifications. For details, contact the Special Sales Department, Skyhorse Publishing, 307 West 36th Street, 11th Floor, New York, NY 10018 or info@skyhorsepublishing.com.

Skyhorse® and Skyhorse Publishing® are registered trademarks of Skyhorse Publishing, Inc.®, a Delaware corporation.

Visit our website at www.skyhorsepublishing.com.

10 9 8 7 6 5 4 3 2 1

Library of Congress Cataloging-in-Publication Data is available on file.

Book and cover design by Liz Price-Kellogg & Kristen Taylor

Front cover, back cover, and interior photography by Blake Price-Kellogg, Liz Price-Kellogg, Jonathan Taylor & Kristen Taylor

Print ISBN: 978-1-63450-351-8
Ebook ISBN: 978-1-5107-0118-2

Printed in China

FOR THE LOVE OF FOOD AND YOGA

Skyhorse Publishing books may be purchased in bulk at special discounts for sales promotion, corporate gifts, fund-raising, or educational purposes. Special editions can also be created to specifications. For details, contact the Special Sales Department, Skyhorse Publishing, 307 West 36th Street, 11th Floor, New York, NY 10018 or info@skyhorsepublishing.com.

Skyhorse® and Skyhorse Publishing® are registered trademarks of Skyhorse Publishing, Inc.®, a Delaware corporation.

Visit our website at www.skyhorsepublishing.com.

10 9 8 7 6 5 4 3 2 1

Library of Congress Cataloging-in-Publication Data is available on file.

Book and cover design by Liz Price-Kellogg & Kristen Taylor

Front cover, back cover, and interior photography by Blake Price-Kellogg, Liz Price-Kellogg, Jonathan Taylor & Kristen Taylor

Print ISBN: 978-1-63450-351-8
Ebook ISBN: 978-1-5107-0118-2

Printed in China

FOR THE LOVE OF FOOD AND YOGA

A CELEBRATION OF MINDFUL EATING AND BEING

**LIZ PRICE-KELLOGG
& KRISTEN TAYLOR**

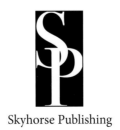

Skyhorse Publishing

REMARKS

"This is a wonderful book, all about mindful living, eating, and being. Through recipes and photographs taken in one of the most beautiful places in North America, *For the Love of Food and Yoga* demonstrates just how thrilling the journey can be."

Jennifer Trainer Thompson, Author of more than sixteen books, including *Jump Up and Kiss Me: Spicy Vegetarian Cooking*, and three-time James Beard Foundation Awards Nominee

"Such a refreshing way to look at and experience the 'yoga' of eating … Beautiful pictures of places, poses, people, and plates of healthy, vibrant food. The book is sprinkled with subtle humor on literally every page, along with recipes just inviting us back to our kitchens to prepare and enjoy with friends and family. What a concept!"

Peter Sterios, ERYT-500, Creator of Manduka & Creator of *Gravity & Grace* DVDs

"*For the Love of Food and Yoga* is a feast for the eyes, palate, body and soul. Liz and Kristen share their authentic way of living with us. Their book will leave you feeling enriched and inspired."

Katrin J. Schubert, MD, PhD, Author of the *5 Minute First Aid for the Mind* series

"The combination of inspirational quotes, thoughtful writing, creative recipes, and photographs of asanas set within the beauty of the natural environment encourages us to take a deeper and more conscious approach to nourishing our bodies and feeding our souls. This book is an important addition to any yoga practitioner's library."

Kathy Falge, MA, LMT, KPJAYI Authorized Level 2 Ashtanga Yoga Teacher

FOREWORD

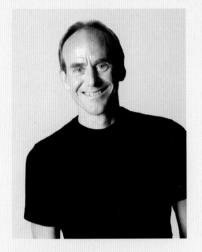

David Swenson

As David Swenson says, *"There's magic in the minutiae."*

The mood is in the food! This adage I truly believe. A good meal is tasted not only with the tongue but also with our eyes, our sense of smell, and even our soul. Those that enjoy the process of preparing a meal, presenting it with grace, and relishing seeing others gain joy, strength, and nourishment from their creations are true artists. In the pages of their book: *For the Love of Food and Yoga*, Liz and Kristen have proven that they are truly such artistic souls. They have captured in exquisite photography succulent and tantalizing dishes with simple–to-follow recipes for nutritious, conscious meals and snacks. With catchy names like the Cobbler's Kale Chips and Holy Guacamole, they keep it fun and interesting. The interspersion of yoga asanas, inspirational quotations, and thoughtful yogic writings provides a wonderful representation of the holistic web of the food we eat, the thoughts we think, and the paths we tread. Enjoy your journey through the book. You are sure to come out the other end with not only some great recipes and a satisfied palate, but potentially new insights and awareness of the true meaning of Yoga as Union or Balance within all realms of life.

David Swenson is recognized today as one of the world's foremost practitioners and instructors of Ashtanga yoga. David began practicing yoga at a very early age. He made his first trip to Mysore, India in 1977 and learned the full Ashtanga system as it was originally taught by Sri K. Pattabhi Jois. David is the author of *Ashtanga Yoga: The Practice Manual*, a celebrated, world-renowned, instructional book that has been translated in several languages.

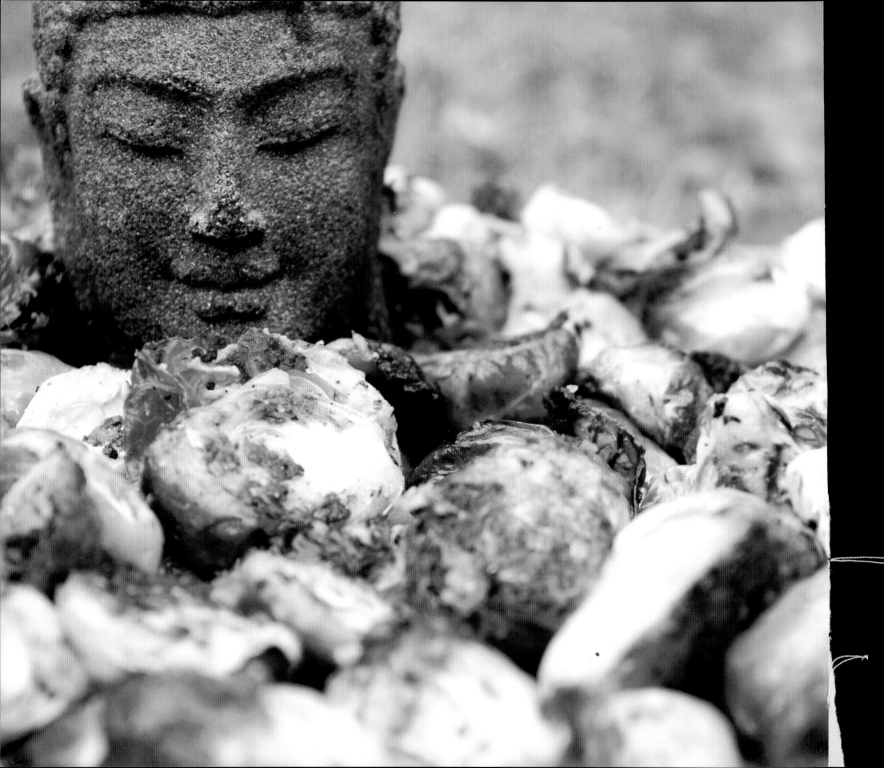

TABLE OF CONTENTS

ABOUT LIZ

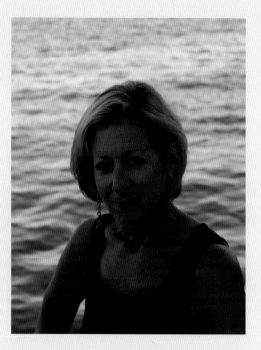

My first yoga class, nearly twenty years ago, felt like an awakening. That class, with yoga teacher Linda Kaplan, left me feeling sweaty, exhausted, exhilarated, and with an undeniable sense of clarity. In my first year of regular practice, Linda's advice and mantra—"do more yoga"—lead to an enlightenment beyond just strengthening the body and calming the mind. My practice began to trickle down into the most mundane tasks, often making them effortless and even enjoyable. Since that time, my mat has become a place of honesty, simplicity, mindfulness, and discovery.

That my yoga practice would transcend into my food choices and food experiences was inevitable. I had begun my vegetarian journey in my teens and was committed to raising a strong, healthy family—including my children, Taylor and Blake, and husband, Jeremy—with natural and wholesome food choices. My yoga practice, however, helped me to cultivate a *loving* relationship with food. In a culture that seems simultaneously obsessed with overeating and dieting, a more effective approach—from my mat to yours—is to be yourself, be mindful, listen to your body, celebrate your food and its inherent benefits, and be grateful!

For almost two decades I have been the "caregiver" for *River Yoga*, a responsibility that brings me great joy as it enables me to continually learn from my students and celebrate their unique practices. I grew up in Skaneateles, New York, and studied fine arts at *St. Lawrence University* and *Syracuse University*. My Ashtanga yoga teacher training began with David Swenson, and I received my Hatha yoga certification from Temple of Kriya Yoga in Chicago, Illinois. This book would not have come to fruition without my writing partner Kristen's enthusiasm and fierce determination. In addition to her being an invaluable friend, yoga student, and guru in her own right, she is a masterful, if not magical, wordsmith. It is my hope that our journey together—as we share our recipes, insights, and stories of *food* and *yoga*—will encourage and inspire your own.

ABOUT KRISTEN

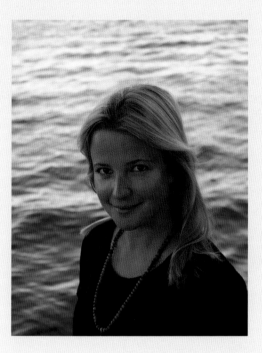

My *aha!* yoga moment didn't happen overnight. In the light of authenticity, I admit that I took my first few yoga classes because I wanted the "yoga body." And, quite frankly, because exercise and achieving a certain body ideal were the goals, I didn't initially embrace yoga. Then, I found my teacher, Liz, and something huge clicked. Liz provided me with an extraordinary foundation to explore and celebrate the ancient teachings of yoga and to find my unique yogic path. What I have learned from Liz and my yoga practice, thus far, has been completely life changing. Yoga continues to be an ever-present part of my life. It helps me to find stillness, feel gratitude, be present, and create stronger connections with family, friends, my community, and food.

As I developed my yoga practice, I also developed my vegetarian lifestyle. I slowly introduced vegetarian and vegan meals into my daily diet. As a result, I became increasingly aware of how the foods I ate affected how I thought and felt. I also realized I didn't need to eat meat to sustain a balanced, nutritious diet, and felt a connection to following the yoga teachings of *ahimsa*, or non-harming. Embracing a predominantly plant-based diet has brought more ease and joy into my kitchen. It has also helped to shift my focus from eating to satiate hunger or maintain a certain weight to eating to feel healthy and energized. Choosing foods that strengthen and empower my body and mind has become an integral, and even effortless component of my path toward whole health. Creating and cooking delicious, simple, and flavorful vegetarian food has become one of my biggest passions.

I live with my family—including my children, Grace and Max, and husband, Jon—in the Thousand Islands, New York. This is a majestic place, which I thank for its unique and beautiful inspirations. I grew up in State College, Pennsylvania, and studied communications at *The George Washington University* in Washington, D.C. I have thoroughly enjoyed and learned so much from co-creating this book. Thankfully, the lessons keep coming.

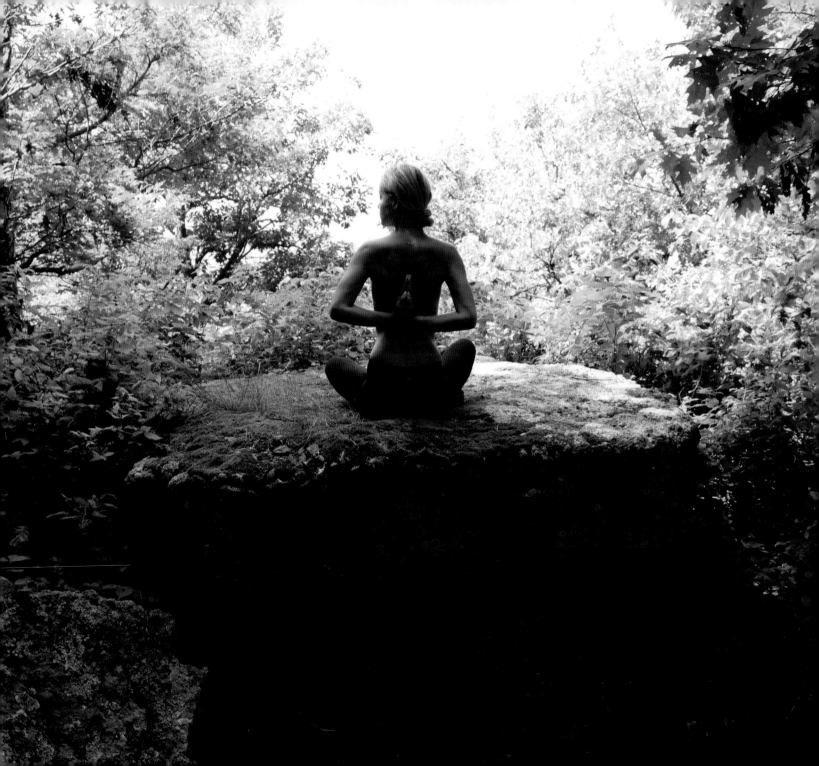

GRATITUDE

"The attitude of gratitude is the highest yoga."
YOGI BHAJAN

This book is dedicated to the love of food, yoga, and . . . you. Below we would like to also thank individuals and places in our past and present that have contributed to the shape of our lives—who and where we are—and, subsequently, this book. Thank you. Namaste.

Alex & BJ Mosher; Andrea Dick; Angie Hegazi; Ann Spurrell & Family; Ariana "Zaza" Carpenter & Family; Barbara Morar & Family; Beverly & The Messenger-Harris Family; Blake Price-Kellogg; Brandon & Team Ream; Carol Kellogg Clarke; Carrie French & Family; Carrie Schneider; Casie Renfrew & Family; Childhood Friendships; Crystal Amo; Cynthia Matthews & Family; Dan "Dad" LeKander; David Swenson; Debra Newman; Deepak Chopra; Ed Grocholski; Emily Costantino; Family; Fred "PapPap" Hall & The Hall Family; George Houghton; Ginny Scoles & Family; Glo Reinman; Grace Taylor; Grambo, Deb and The Kellogg Family; Gramma Selner; Jennifer Cring; Jennifer Trainer Thompson; Jeremy Kellogg; Jackie Humilovich & Family; Jodi Butler & Family; Jonathan Lorin Taylor; Kate Lorenz; Kathy Sommer; Katrin Schubert; Kay "Mom" Price; Kelly French & Family; Kim Schwartz; "Loveee" Dombrowski & Family; Lynn Taylor & Family; Mary & The Taylor Family; Max Taylor; Monica, Mana & The Behan Family; Nancy Chambers Aubertine & Family; Nathan Whittaker; Nellie & Steve Taylor; Oprah Winfrey; Our Community; Our Teachers; Pearly; Peggy "Mom" LeKander; Peter Purcell; Peter Sterios; Phyllis Gardner; Rick Moore; River Yoga Students (Past, Present and Future) & Teachers (Linda Kaplan, Jules Flora, Laura Cerow, Lisa Tiffany, Stephanie Moon, Trisha Crowe, Julia Bonisteel, Kathy Falge, Mary Brownell, Dory Sheldon, Kara Healy, Kelli Gould, Eliza Moore, Andy Greene, and Lori Arnot); Roger Lindberg; Sally & Cherie; Sarah Purcell; Susan Bach; Susan Murray Lyon & Family; Suzanne, Momcat and The Haux Nest; Sheri & The Buchen Family; Susan McClennen Phear & Family; Taylor Price-Kellogg; The Chase Family; The Fletcher Family; The Fulmer Family; The Gefell Families; The Purcell Family; Thousand Islands (New York); Tiffany Barsotti; Tracy Kurtenbach; Uncy Bill & Herb Usher; Wendy "Mimi" Thompson PhD & Family; Win Price & Family; Windsor "Dad" Price; Vicky & Jay Gilbert

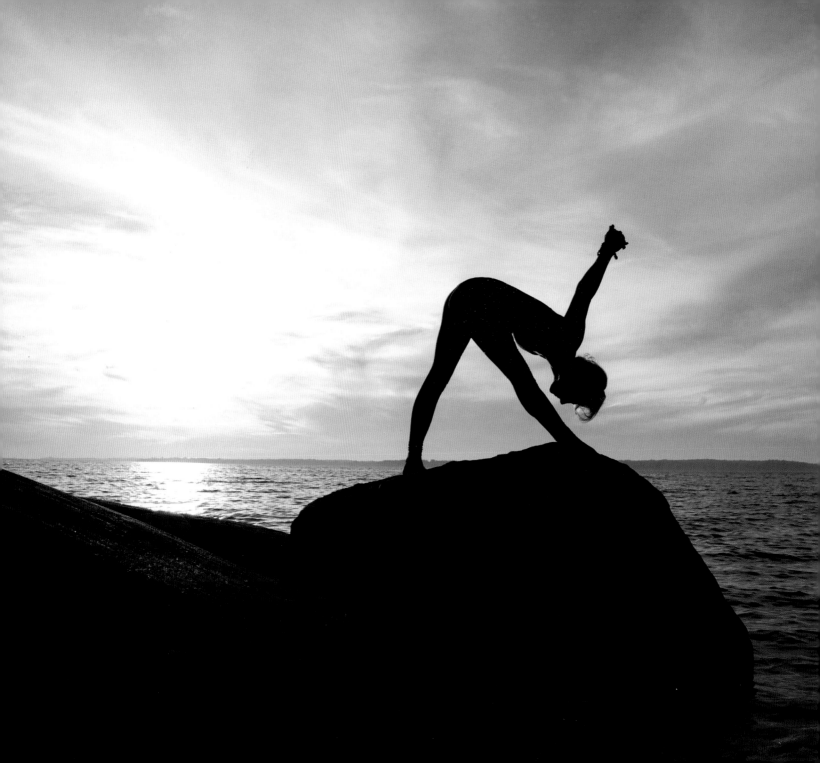

A GREETING

Welcome!

For the Love of Food and Yoga: A Celebration of Mindful Eating and Being is an exploration of how the inner awareness we develop on our yoga mats fuels our bodies, minds, and overall states of wellbeing, which subsequently influences our lifestyles and food experiences. We believe the lessons that are integral to the practice of yoga—*mindfulness, presence, intention, gratitude,* and *joy*—are also fully present in the practices of living, cooking, and eating well.

The practice of yoga—postures and breath—is a vehicle to awaken and embolden the inherent connection between mind, body, and inner spirit. Though yoga is an exercise for the body, it is more importantly an exercise for the mind that builds a pathway for self-improvement. Yoga is a bouquet of life lessons available for the taking. The practice of yoga is a journey, an evolution, and a way of life.

Through our yoga practices, we become more aware about how we feel on a deeper level. Yoga embraces the consumption of simple, natural, and wholesome foods that promote good health. There is an opportunity for the purchasing, preparation, and enjoyment of food to be mindful, present, joyful, and delicious by utilizing all of our senses *and* sensibility. It is in this state of aware eating that we are able to develop an even healthier being—physically, mentally, and spiritually. The pursuit of conscious consumption is ultimately addictive as we end up feeling better and better about ourselves.

Your commitment to self discovery through yoga and mindful eating takes effort and dedication. *Breathe. Laugh.* Trust the path that you are on, including those moments or experiences you may perceive to be triumphs or failures. A practice should not be the exact same every time. The same ingredients may not be available all of the time, just as certain postures and flexibility may not be available to you from one yoga practice to the next. Accept who you are and what you have in the present.

Our book is presented through a joyful compilation of one hundred time-tested yoga teachings—"YogiBites"—married with one hundred delicious, common sense vegetarian, vegan, or raw recipes. The recipes and teachings outlined in the book should be used with modifications and variations to fit where you are in your life or your practice. Our intention is for all of us to learn from the student and teacher within as we celebrate our practices, delicious meals, time with friends and family, and those (seemingly) small happenings.

As with all food choices, take it with a grain of salt. And, bless your mess.

Namaste,

Liz & Kristen

RECIPES

"By the purity of food, follows the purification of the inner nature."
SWAMI SIVANANDA

As our yoga practices support our physical, mental, emotional, and spiritual health, a yogic diet is typically vegetarian because it promotes a healthy body and mind and is in accord with the yogic path toward spiritual wellbeing. We have included one hundred of our favorite simple, delicious, and nutritionally packed recipes in this book. We encourage you to use all of your senses and sensibility (common sense) when choosing and eating foods, making modifications or variations to recipes as necessary based on what is fresh, organic, and local. As we promote flexibility in our yoga practices, we think it is important to offer "flexible recipes." All of our recipes are vegetarian, vegan or vegan optional *(v)*, or raw or raw optional *(r)*. Please make adjustments to fit your practice (and pantry). Enjoy!

YOGIBITES

YogiBites is a collection of celebrated yoga teachings that are presented as postures, philosophies, intentions, quotes, and photos. These are lessons that you may choose to explore on and off of the mat. Keep your eyes and mind open to those special gifts that awaken the connection between mind, body, and inner spirit.

- YOGA
- PRACTICE
- CONSCIOUSNESS
- GRATITUDE
- Phalakasana / Plank Pose
- Baddha Konasana / Cobbler's Pose
- MEDITATION
- Uttana Padasana / Extended Leg Fish Pose
- AHIMSA
- Urdhva Dhanurasana / Full Wheel or Upward Facing Bow Pose
- BREATH
- PRESENCE
- BE
- HAPPY
- DEDICATIONS
- ABUNDANCE
- COMMON SENSE
- MEDICINE CABINET
- SILENCE
- WISDOM
- Vrksasana I / Tree Pose
- BALANCE
- Utkatasana / Chair Pose
- Salamba Sirsasana / Supported Headstand
- CREATE
- JOY
- RESPONSIBILITY
- GROWTH
- Urdhva Pavanamuktasana / Standing Wind Relieving or Knee-to-Chest Pose
- Vrschikasana / Scorpion

- THE RIVER YOGA COMMUNITY
- HARMONY
- INTENTION INGREDIENTS
- INTENTION / ATTENTION
- COURAGE
- KARMA
- FREEDOM
- ENERGY
- Virasana / Hero Pose
- Ardha Matsyendrasana / Half Lord of the Fishes Pose
- LOVE
- Ananda Balasana / Happy Baby Pose
- FEARLESSNESS
- Utkata Konasana / Goddess Pose
- SWAMI VIVEKANANDA: FOLLOW YOUR YELLOW BRICK ROAD
- FULFILLMENT
- SIMPLICITY
- PATIENCE
- Bhujangasana / Cobra Pose
- CONFIDENCE
- PARTNER
- FRIENDSHIP
- VEGETARIANISM
- MINDFULNESS
- HOME
- Ardha Chandrasana I / Half Moon Pose
- Parivrtta Trikonasana / Revolved Triangle Pose
- FLEXIBILITY
- ACTION
- Viparita Virabhadrasana / Exalted Warrior Pose
- Padmasana / Lotus Posture

- SAVOR
- Navasana / Boat Pose
- EFFORT
- Halasana / Plough Pose
- Utthita Parsvakonasana III / Advanced Extended Side Angle Pose
- Setu Bandhasana / Bridge Pose
- CONTENTMENT (SANTOSA)
- Balasana / Child's Pose
- TRANSITION
- SURRENDER
- WASHING THE DISHES TO WASH THE DISHES
- Tadasana / Mountain Pose
- Parsva Bhuja Dandasana / Grasshopper
- PASSION
- Trikonasana / Triangle Pose
- Anjali Mudra / Hand Gesture with Namaste or Prayer Seal
- PURPOSE
- GRACE
- POWER

- BLISS
- DREAM
- AWARENESS
- Salamba Sarvangasana / Supported Shoulderstand
- Svarga Dvijasana / Bird of Paradise
- Urdhva Prasarita Eka Padasana / Standing Split
- Hanumanasana / Monkey God Posture
- NATURE
- HUMILITY
- Savasana / Corpse Pose
- CELEBRATE
- PLAY
- Eka Pada Galavasana / Flying Crow
- Urdhva Mukha Svanasana / Upward Facing Dog Pose
- Bakasana / Crow
- EXPLORE
- Ardha Ustrasana / Half Camel Posture
- Natarajasana III / Advanced King Dancer
- HEALING
- SPIRITUALITY

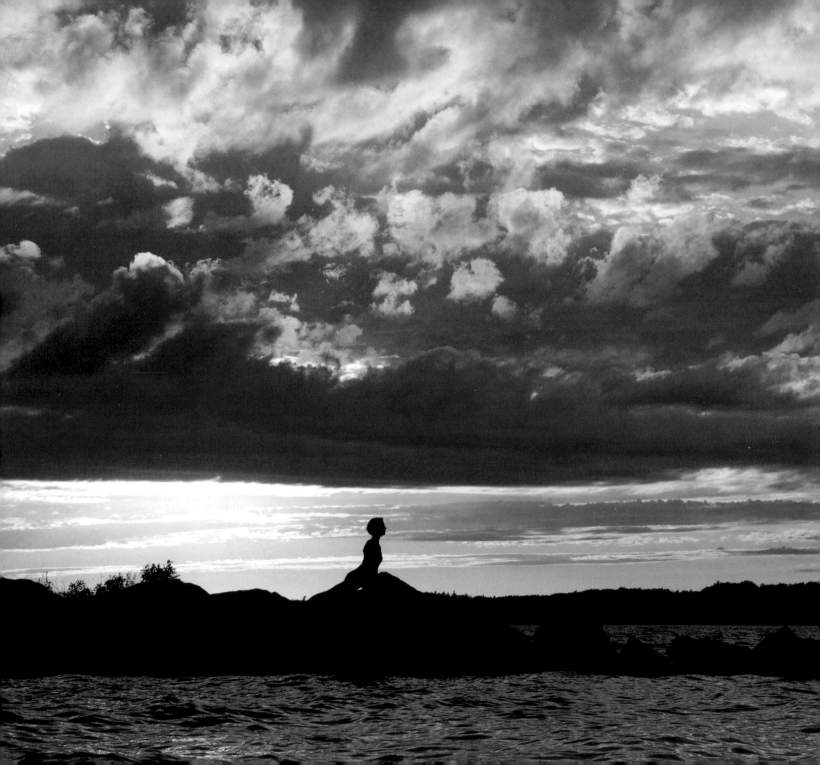

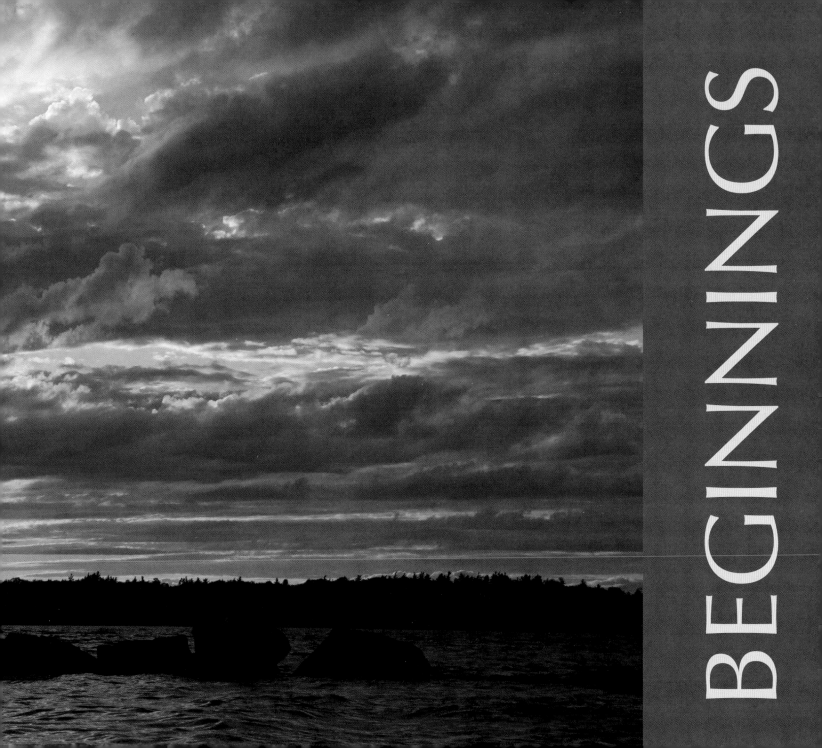

BEGINNINGS

YOGA

"You cannot do yoga. Yoga is your natural state. What you can do are yoga exercises, which may reveal to you where you are resisting your natural state."
SHARON GANNON

Yoga, meaning "union," is an ancient science and practice of exploring and nurturing the inherent connection between mind, body, and inner spirit. Yoga teaches us to look inward and focus on the breath, *pranayama*, and that in the stillness of being, we are able to find a deeper sense of awareness. Through the physical practice of yoga postures, or *asanas*, we become aware of any areas of tightness or resistance in the body. This offers an opportunity to strengthen, energize, calm, and open the physical body, and ultimately, the mind. Yoga enables us to concentrate on the intention of our thoughts and actions with the ultimate goal of unveiling and celebrating our own true nature.

The awareness we develop through our yoga practices may transcend to, and influence, all aspects of our lives—including our lifestyles and food experiences. Awareness is the first and most important step in choosing foods that will nurture and embolden the body. As we become more conscientious about how the foods we eat affect our overall wellness, we naturally make choices that help us to achieve greater health and prevent "dis-ease."

PRACTICE

"Do your practice and all is coming."
SRI K. PATTABHI JOIS

IT IS YOUR PRACTICE. Through our yoga and eating practices we have an opportunity to be mindful of where we are in the present. Our practices, however, are not limited to our mats or our kitchens. Leading Western Ashtanga yoga teacher, David Swenson, says our practices serve as a "healing balm for the rest of our lives." Practice takes effort and dedication, but it should not feel like a chore. Celebrate the process and explore the subtleties of your present state. Remember that your current state is not permanent. It is simply part of the journey.

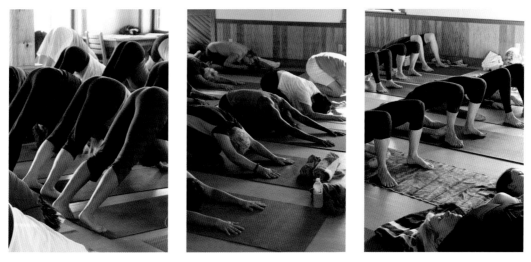

T.I. Park Pavilion River Yoga Class

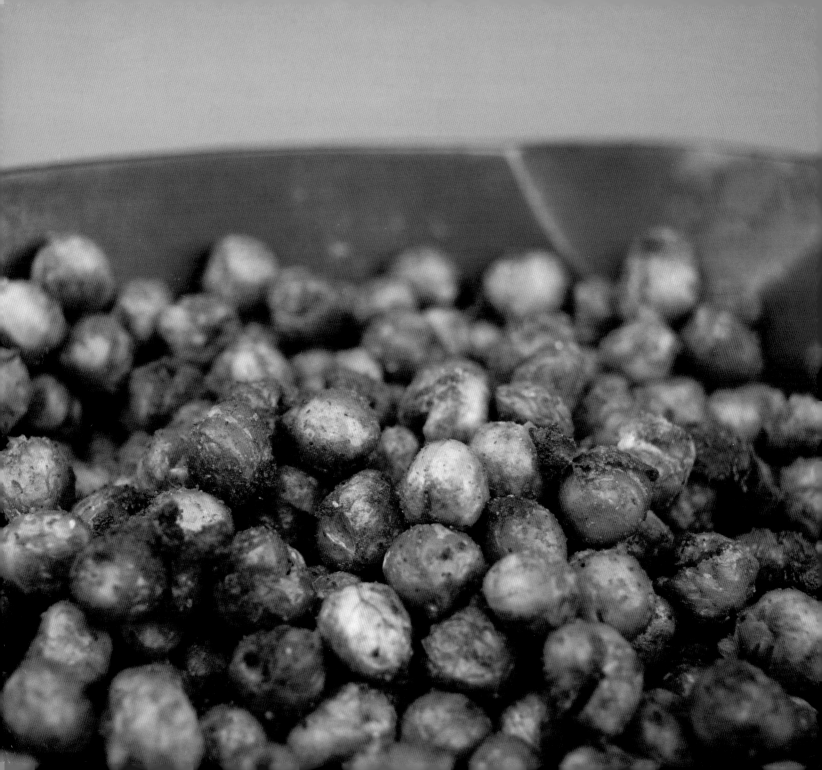

CONSCIOUS CHICKS *(v)*

Each "Conscious Chicks" variation offers a unique flavor experience and is easy to prepare. Chickpeas, known formally as garbanzo beans, are a great source of protein, iron, and manganese, which aids in energy production. Conscious Chicks may be served as an appetizer or as a side dish. Not-So-Plain Chicks, Curry Chicks, and Smokin' Chicks are great substitutes for croutons on salads. Goat Cheesy Chicks are delicious when used as filling for lettuce wraps or as a topping over mixed greens or whole grain pasta. We have offered using canned legumes and beans for ease of preparation and use; however, when preparing legumes and beans throughout the book, please remember to use modifications and variations to fit your lifestyle. Thus, if you would rather start with dried varieties, please do so and adjust the recipes accordingly. Each recipe serves 6–8.

NOT-SO-PLAIN CHICKS & SMOKIN' CHICKS *(v)*

15 oz. canned chickpeas
Himalayan salt and pepper (to taste)
½ tsp. (heaping) smoked paprika (for SMOKIN' CHICKS only)
2T olive oil

1. Preheat oven to 400°F.
2. Rinse and drain chickpeas.
3. Combine chickpeas with remaining ingredients in bowl.
4. Pour onto baking sheet and shake ingredients into a flat layer.
5. Bake for 20 minutes. Then check and shake chickpeas and add salt and/or pepper if needed. Cook for an additional 15 minutes or until chickpeas look crisped but not dried out. Remove from oven and serve warm.

CURRY CHICKS *(v)*

15 oz. canned chickpeas
1 tsp. (heaping) curry powder
Himalayan salt and pepper (to taste)
2T olive oil
½ cup dried, unsweetened cherries
½ cup (loosely packed) cilantro (lightly chopped)

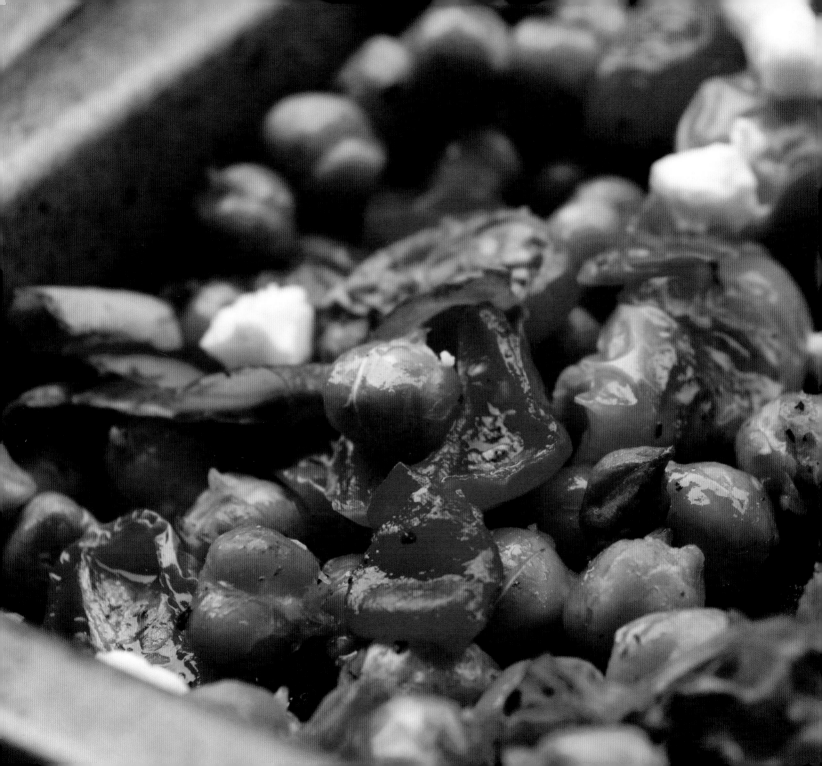

1. Preheat oven to 400°F.
2. Rinse and drain chickpeas.
3. Combine chickpeas with curry powder, salt, pepper, and olive oil in bowl.
4. Pour onto baking sheet and shake ingredients into a flat layer.
5. Bake for 20 minutes. Then check and shake chickpeas and add salt and/or pepper if needed. Cook for an additional 15 minutes or until chickpeas look crisped but not dried out. Remove from oven.
6. Place chickpeas in a bowl or serving dish and mix in cherries and cilantro. Serve warm.

GOAT CHEESY CHICKS

15 oz. canned chickpeas
Himalayan salt and pepper (to taste)
2T olive oil
1 cup cherry tomatoes (halved lengthwise)
½ cup fresh basil leaves (chopped)
1 oz. crumbled goat cheese (optional)

1. Preheat oven to 400°F.
2. Rinse and drain chickpeas.
3. Combine chickpeas with salt, pepper, olive oil, and tomatoes in bowl.
4. Pour onto baking sheet and shake ingredients into a flat layer.
5. Bake for 20 minutes. Then check and shake chickpeas and add salt and/or pepper if needed. Cook for an additional 20 minutes or until chickpeas look crisped but not dried out. Remove from oven.
6. Place cooked mixture in a bowl or serving dish and mix in basil and goat cheese. Serve warm.

CONSCIOUSNESS

"A human being is a part of the whole called by us universe, a part limited in time and space. He experiences himself, his thoughts and feeling as something separated from the rest, a kind of optical delusion of his consciousness. This delusion is a kind of prison for us, restricting us to our personal desires and to affection for a few persons nearest to us. Our task must be to free ourselves from this prison by widening our circle of compassion to embrace all living creatures and the whole of nature in its beauty."
ALBERT EINSTEIN

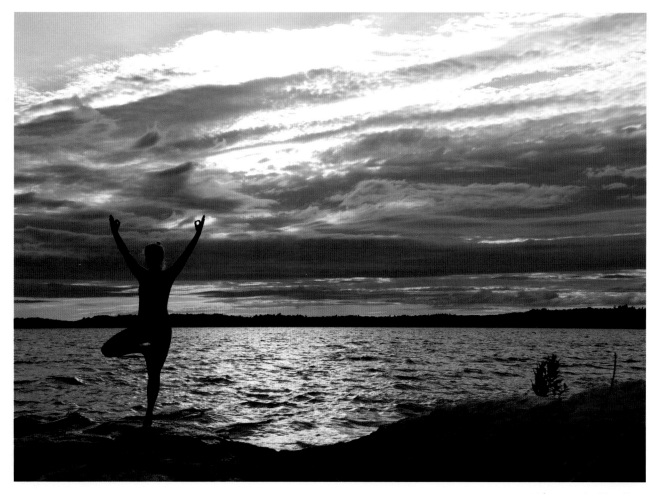

Vrksasana I • Tree Pose

GRATITUDE

"Just for today do not worry. Just for today do not anger. Honor your parents, teachers, and elders. Earn your living honestly. Show gratitude to everything."
DR. MIKAO USUI

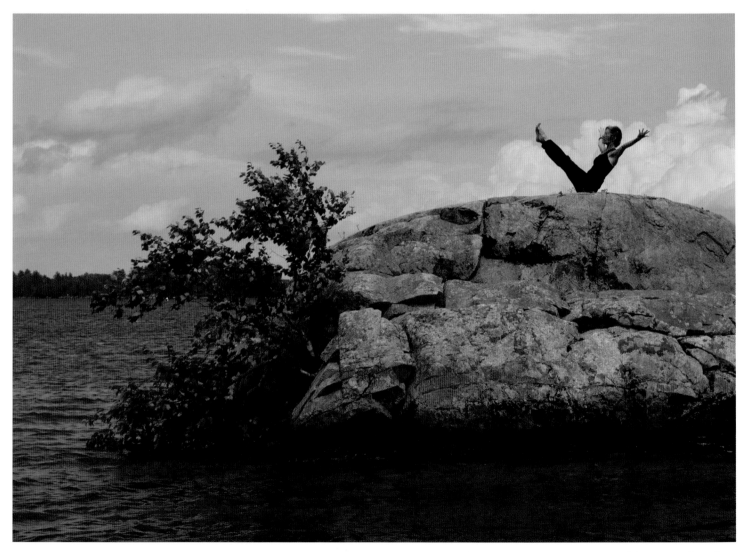

Navasana • Boat Pose

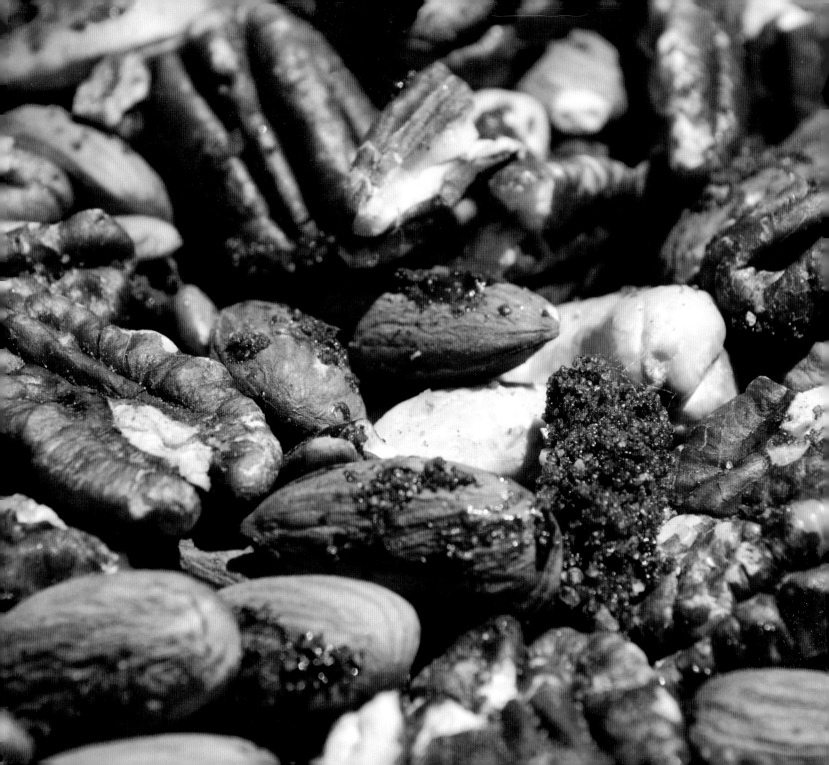

VIGOR NUTS (v)

Our Vigor Nuts are invigorating and nutritious. Eating a variety of nuts, in moderation, provides a variety of health benefits including reducing stress, reducing the risk of heart disease, and aiding in weight maintenance. Modification: Use less (or more) cayenne pepper depending on your desired heat index. Variation: Substitute nuts for other varieties as per your taste preferences. Serves 8–10.

    1 cup raw almonds
    1 cup raw pecan halves
    1 cup raw cashews
    ½ cup pepitas (pumpkin seeds)
    Himalayan salt coarsely ground (to taste)
    Pepper coarsely ground (to taste)
    2 tsp. ground smoked paprika
    ½ tsp. ground cayenne pepper
    3T brown sugar

1. Preheat oven to 350°F.
2. Hand-mix nuts.
3. Combine seasonings in a small bowl.
4. Coat nuts in seasonings. Mix well.
5. Pour nuts onto lightly greased baking sheet and shake into an even layer. Roast for 15 minutes (do not burn). Allow nuts to cool slightly. Serve warm.

PHALAKASANA
PLANK POSE

invigorating, supports bone health, energizing, strengthening, aligning, foundational

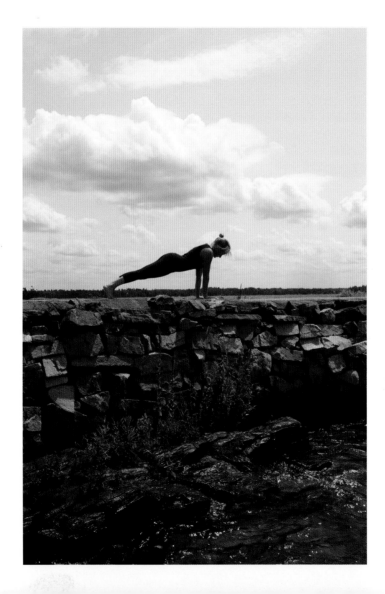

BADDHA KONASANA
COBBLER'S POSE

stimulates circulation, opens hips, soothing, therapeutic

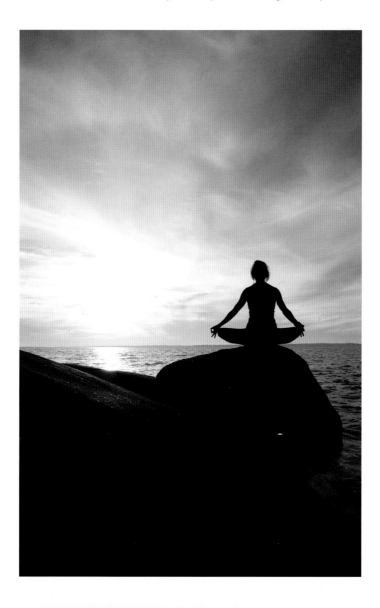

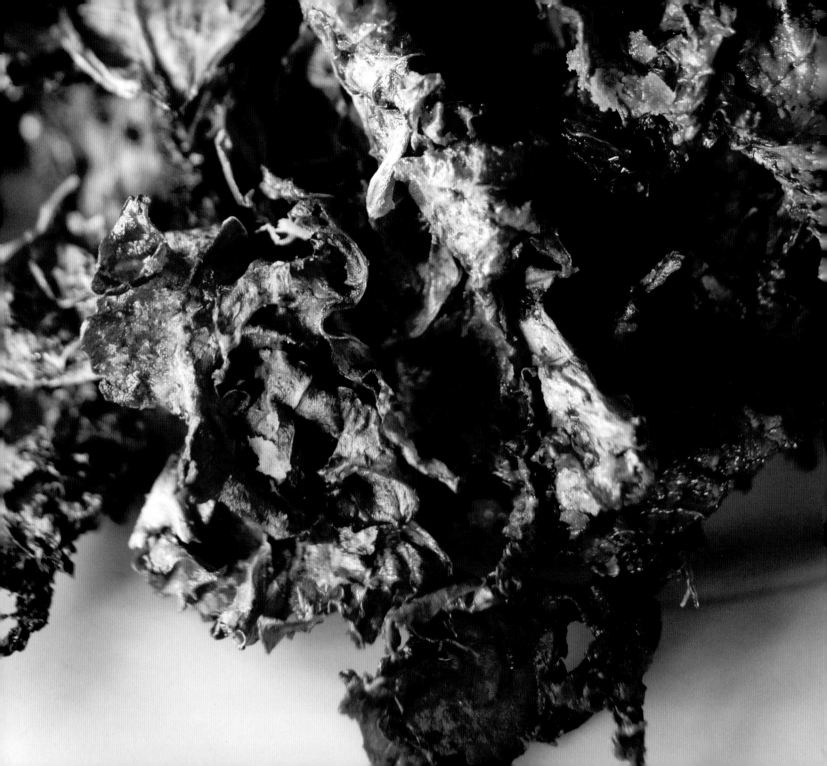

COBBLER'S KALE CHIPS *(v)*

Kale is a "superfood" as it boasts a bevy of health benefits—it is packed with iron, which helps to transport oxygen to various parts of the body, and is also high in calcium, which is good for our bone health and also may be relaxing. Nutritional yeast is a deactivated yeast that is packed with vitamins and protein. It also adds a cheesy flavor to our Cobbler's Kale Chips. This is a delicious, healthy snack that offers an intense flavor and crunch sensation. Serves 4.

1 large bunch of kale (about 4 cups)
4 medium garlic cloves (pressed)
2T olive oil
Himalayan salt coarsely ground (to taste)
Dash of ground cayenne pepper
4T nutritional yeast

1. Preheat oven to 350°F.
2. Wash and thoroughly dry kale. De-rib kale by tearing it off of large stalks and into 2-inch pieces.
3. Toss kale with garlic, olive oil, salt, and cayenne.
4. Pour mixture onto baking sheet and spread into a single layer. Sprinkle evenly with nutritional yeast.
5. Bake for about 20 minutes. Turn kale chips and bake for another 20 minutes or until crisp. Remove and allow to cool.
6. Serve at room temperature in a bowl as finger food.

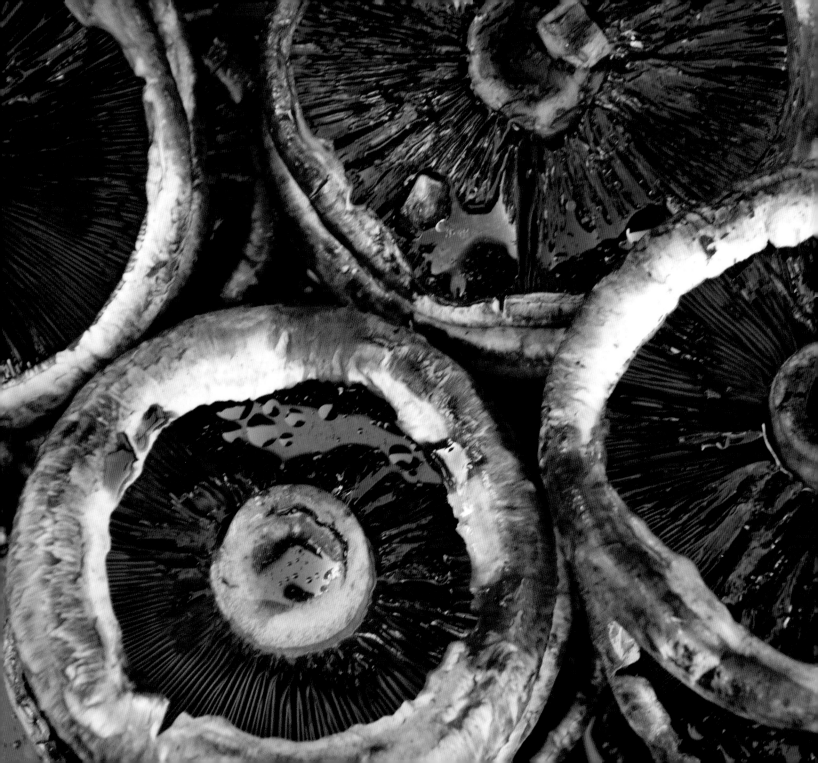

MEDITATIVE MUSHROOMS *(v)*

"Often one goes for one thing and finds another." NEEM KAROLI BABA

We initially thought the "Core Connection" of this recipe would be a wonderful dip; however, upon trying the near-dip recipe, we listened to our instincts and thought it would make an even more sublime stuffing or "core" for a baked Portobello mushroom. And, it does! Thus, with much spontaneity and delight we developed this delicious, healthy stuffed mushroom appetizer, two of which would also make a lovely entrée. Serves 3–6.

Mushrooms
6 large Portobello mushroom caps
2T balsamic vinegar
2T olive oil
1T tamari

Core Connection
¼ cup pine nuts
15 oz. artichoke hearts (in water, drained)
1 cup fresh spinach (loosely packed)
½ cup fresh basil (loosely packed)
7–8 medium fresh cremini mushrooms
4 medium garlic cloves
½ medium white onion
2T lemon juice
6–8T olive oil
Himalayan salt coarsely ground (to taste)
Pepper coarsely ground (to taste)

Garnish
6T Gorgonzola cheese (optional)
Fresh basil leaves

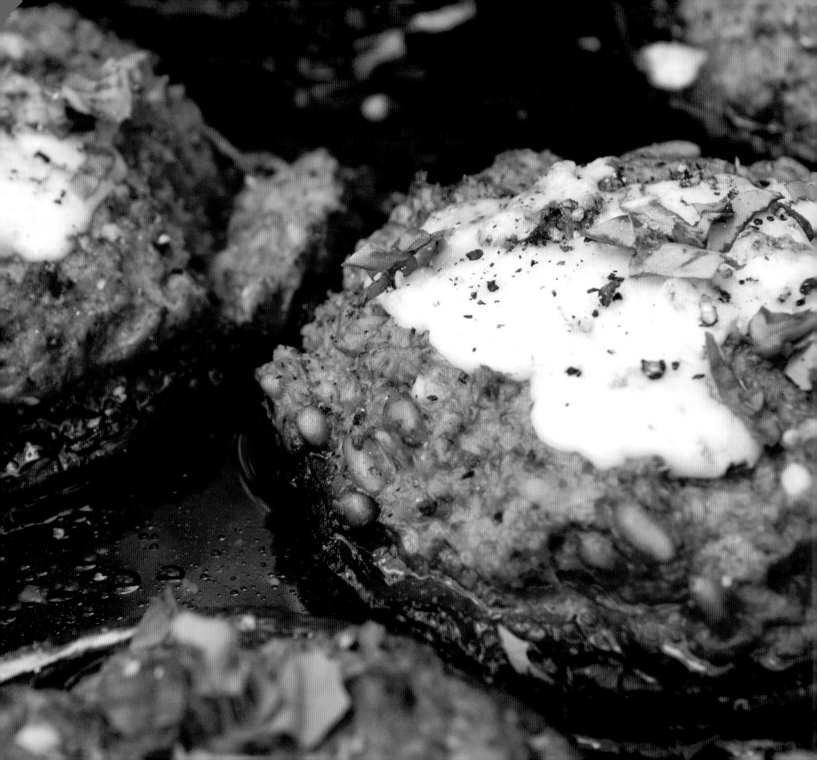

1. Preheat oven to 350°F.
2. Marinate mushroom caps in balsamic vinegar, olive oil, and tamari for 10 to 20 minutes.
3. Toast pine nuts in a medium skillet over low-medium heat until golden brown and fragrant. Remove from heat and set aside.
4. Combine artichokes, spinach, basil, mushrooms, garlic, onion, lemon juice, olive oil, salt, and pepper in food processor, leaving it slightly chunky. Transfer mixture to a bowl and stir in toasted pine nuts.
5. Place marinated mushroom caps on baking sheet. Discard excess marinade.
6. Stuff mushroom caps with *Core Connection*.
7. Bake for 30 minutes. *(For vegan variation, skip to step 9.)*
8. Remove from oven and top each mushroom with one tablespoon of Gorgonzola cheese. Bake for 4 minutes and then broil mushrooms with cheese for 1 minute.
9. Remove mushrooms from oven. Let mushrooms sit on the baking sheet for 5 minutes. Serve topped with fresh basil.

MEDITATION

"Eating mindfully is a most important practice of meditation."
THICH NHAT HANH

We awaken when we shine inward and find our inner silence. It is here where we do not ask for answers or for what we want to hear; without expectations, we simply listen.

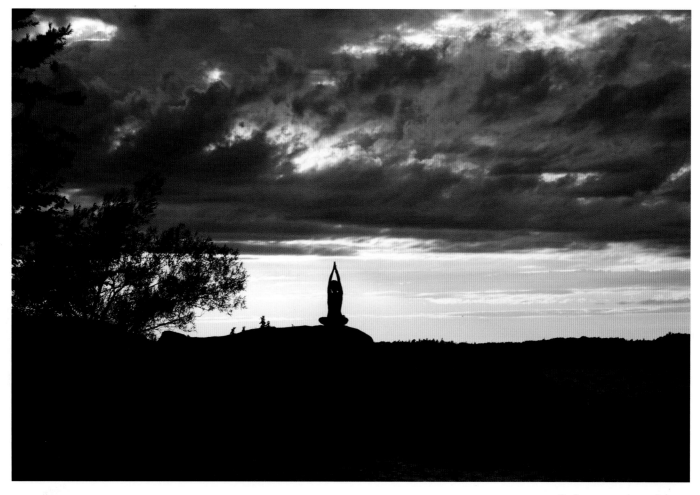

Padmasana • Lotus Posture

UTTANA PADASANA
EXTENDED LEG FISH POSE

*opens the heart center, aids in full breathing, stimulates and
strengthens muscles and organs, improves posture*

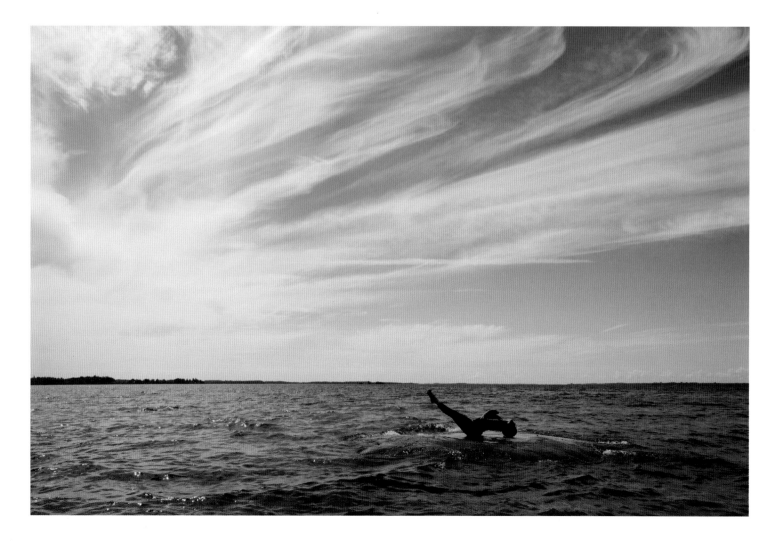

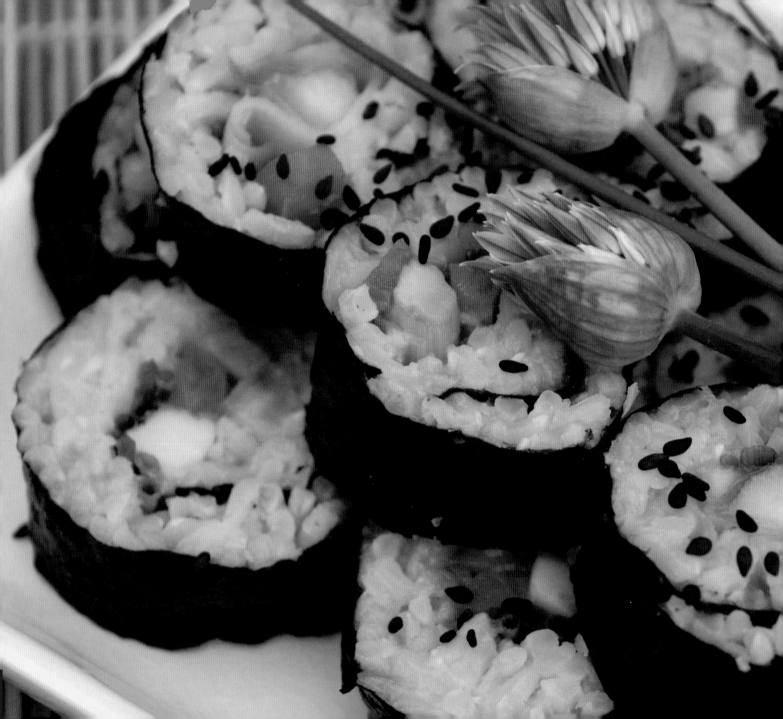

FISH FRIENDLY SUSHI *(v)*

Our Fish Friendly Sushi recipe follows the guidelines of ahimsa, non-harming. *Thus, it contains a variety of nutritionally packed and flavorful vegetables (no fish). It is also served with wasabi and pickled ginger. Wasabi is a Japanese mustard that stimulates the body's natural immune system and is naturally anti-viral, anti-microbial, and anti-bacterial. Ginger is used in many of our recipes. For thousands of years, it has been revered for its therapeutic qualities and also used to help support healthy digestive functioning. Serves 12–14.*

> 2 cups uncooked basmati brown rice
> ½ cup seasoned rice vinegar
> 6 oz. pickled ginger (reserve liquid)
> 6 sheets nori (seaweed sheets)
> 2 cups total of assorted vegetables, julienned or thinly sliced (cucumber, carrot, bell pepper, avocado, asparagus, sprouts, chives, scallions)
> 4T black sesame seeds
> 2T wasabi powder (made into paste with water per package instructions)
> ½ cup tamari (to dip)

1. Cook rice per package instructions. Once rice is cooked, remove from heat. Add rice vinegar and pickled ginger liquid to cooked rice. Set aside and allow to cool. The rice should feel sticky.
2. Place nori, shiny side down, on a horizontally placed sushi mat (you may also use a pliable, non-cloth placemat or plastic wrap).
3. Spread cooked and seasoned rice on top of nori, leaving a 1-inch border at the top edge of the nori sheet.
4. Place ginger and three or four choices of vegetables along a horizontal line, about 2 inches above the bottom edge of the nori.
5. Starting at the bottom edge of your sushi mat, roll the nori sheet away from you, firmly compressing the roll. Wet the exposed nori border at the top to complete your roll.
6. Using a sharp knife, slice rolls into 1-inch rounds. Garnish with sesame seeds and serve with wasabi, pickled ginger, and tamari.

AHIMSA (NON-VIOLENCE)

"I do feel that spiritual progress does demand, at some stage, that we should cease to kill our fellow creatures for the satisfaction of our bodily wants."
MAHATMA GANDHI

Simply, *ahimsa* is the act of kindness and consideration to all beings. In our yoga practices, it speaks to being mindful of our bodies' present strengths and limitations. In our food choices, it speaks to eating healthy, nutritious foods and abstaining from the consumption of animal meats. In our friendships and relationships, it speaks to being open, truthful, and compassionate. In our personal journeys, it speaks to contributing to our own contentment, happiness, and freedom.

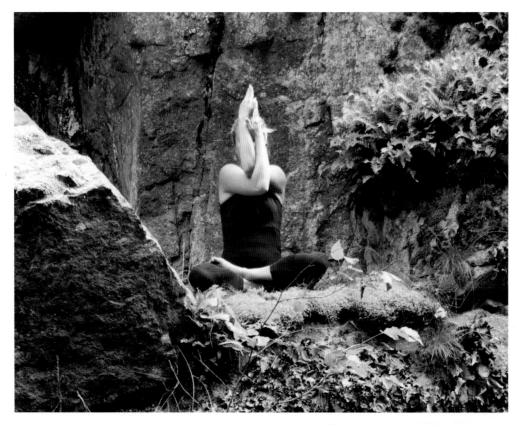

Ardha Padmasana • Half Lotus Posture

URDHVA DHANURASANA
FULL WHEEL OR UPWARD FACING BOW POSE

opens heart center, energizing, strengthening, stimulates thyroid

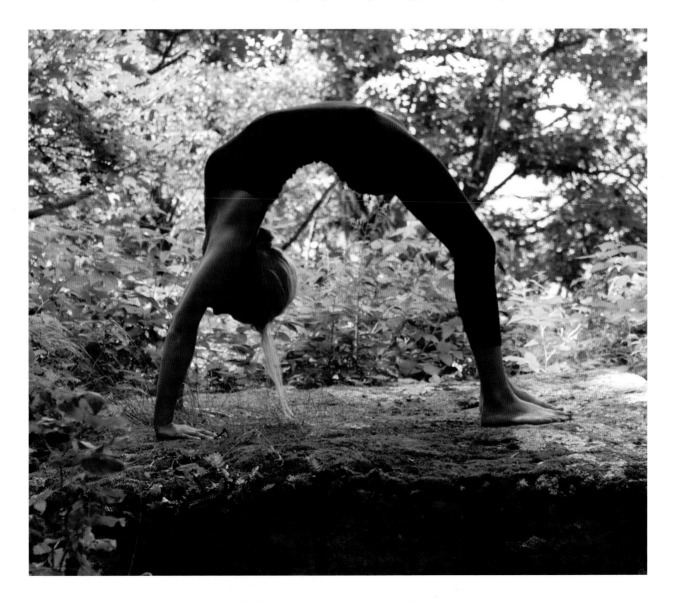

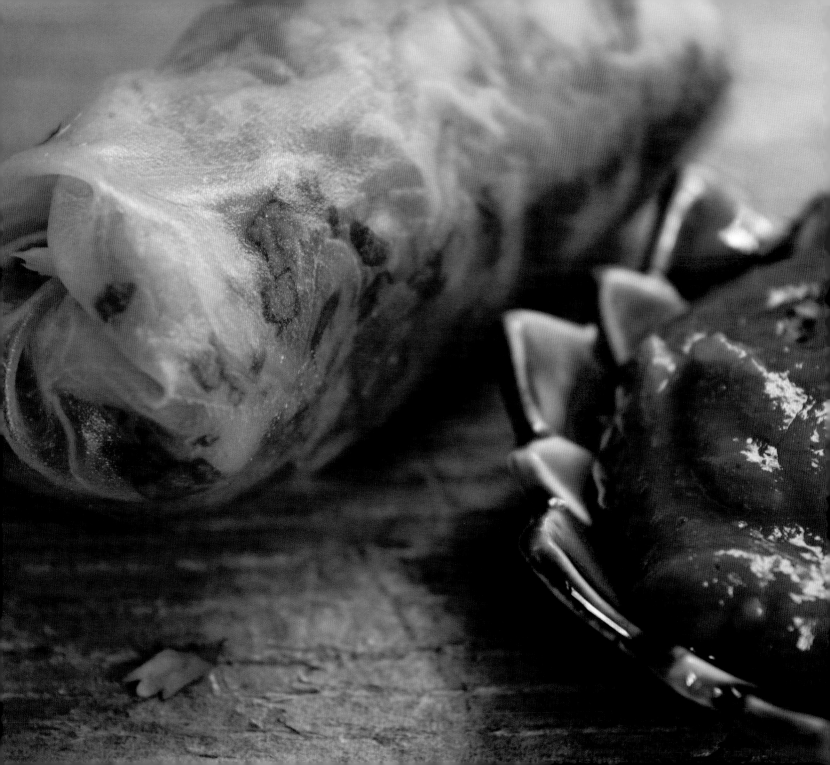

RICE WHEELS (v)

Asian food often bursts with flavor and is effortlessly vegan. Our Rice Wheels are our variation of Vietnamese Summer Rolls and they may be cut into 1-inch rounds to form edible "wheels." The slaw for the Rice Wheels incorporates a traditional Vietnamese Summer Roll dipping sauce, Nuoc Cham, and is also used in The Happy Pig Banh Mi (see recipe on page 176). Serves 4.

Slaw
½ cup seasoned rice vinegar
2T tamari
2T lime juice
1 medium garlic clove (minced)
Red pepper flakes (to taste)
Himalayan salt coarsely ground (to taste)
1 cup carrot (shredded)
1 cup daikon radish (shredded)

Sweetly Spicy Peanut Dipping Sauce
½ cup chunky peanut butter
3T Hoisin sauce
3T lime juice
1T brown sugar

1T chili garlic sauce
1T sesame oil
2T tamari
4T seasoned rice vinegar
1T fresh ginger (minced)
1 medium garlic clove (minced)
¼ cup freshly chopped peanuts (garnish)

Rice paper wrappers (8 large)
1 cup cucumber (thinly sliced on diagonal
   to create skewed rounds)
¼ cup mint (chopped)
¼ cup basil (chopped)
¼ cup cilantro (chopped)

1. Combine rice vinegar, tamari, lime juice, garlic, red pepper flakes, and salt in a medium mixing bowl to create slaw dressing. Once combined, add shredded carrot and daikon. Set aside for at least 30 minutes.
2. Combine all ingredients for Dipping Sauce. Place in four dipping bowls and top equally with chopped peanuts.
3. In a pie dish, soak rice wrappers one at a time in very warm water. Once softened, immediately transfer to paper towel–lined plate. In the center of the wrapper, line up three cucumber slices, overlapping slightly. Next, using a slotted spoon, add one-eighth of the slaw followed by one-eighth of each of the herbs. Fold in the shorter exposed sides of the wrapper, and then roll the wrapper tightly from one of the longer exposed sides of the wrapper to the other. Once a Rice Wheel is complete, place it on plastic wrap. Repeat eight to form eight rolls. Plate with *Dipping Sauce* and serve immediately.

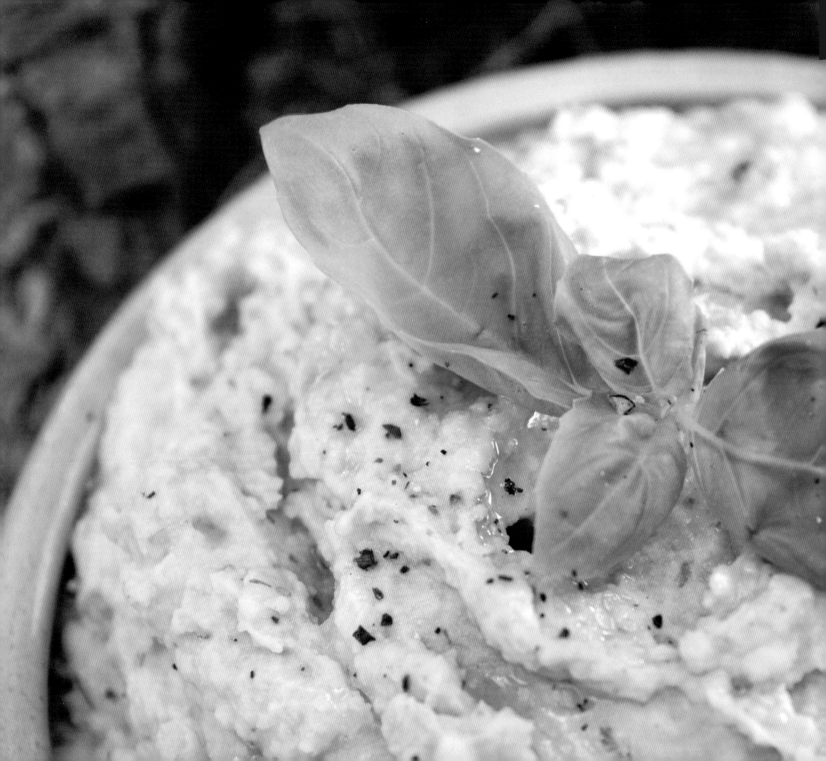

SO HUM . . . MUS *(v)*

The name of this very garlicky, lemony, and delicious hummus recipe is a play on the meditative chant "so hum," which is a reflection of sounding breath (Ujjayi). It helps to focus the mind on a state of unified consciousness. "So" carries the meaning "I am" and "hum" carries the meaning "that"; thus, the chant brings awareness to the belief that "I am that. That I am."

The inclusion of lemon flax seed oil provides omega-3 fatty acids, which reduce risk of cancer, heart disease, stroke, and diabetes. Variation: Add peeled, diced carrots or chopped, seeded red peppers for additional nutritional value and color. As a delightful option, top hummus with Blakey's Balsamic Glaze (see recipe on page 164). Serves 4–8.

15 oz. canned chickpeas (reserve water)
3T lemon juice (at room temperature)
1T olive oil
1T lemon flax seed oil
¼ cup tahini
2T tamari
3 medium garlic cloves (crushed)
Pepper to taste
2T fresh dill (optional)
¼ cup basil (plus more for garnish)

1. Reserve chickpea water. Drain and rinse chickpeas.
2. Combine all ingredients in a food processor and process until creamy. Add reserved chickpea water if needed to reach desired consistency.
3. Serve in a delightful bowl and garnish with basil leaves.

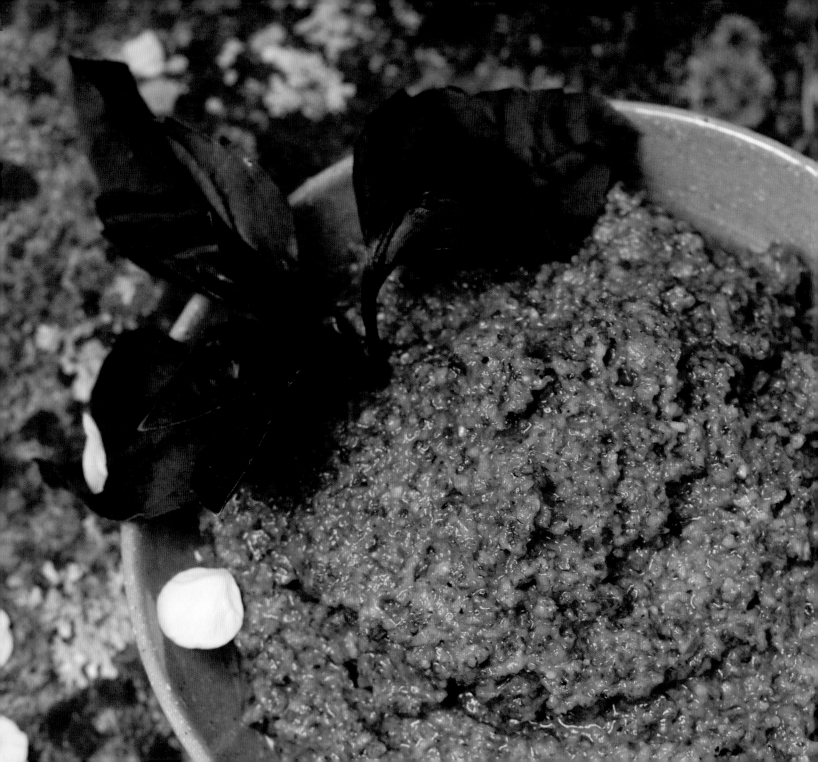

PRANA PESTO *(v)*

In Sanskrit, prana means "life force" or "breath." By regulating our breath, pranayama, we support our physical, mental, and emotional wellbeing. Focus on your breath to become better aware of the joys of cooking and eating. Our Prana Pesto uses pecans instead of pine nuts, which may be more affordable. Variation: Use pine nuts, walnuts, or another nut of your choice. This pesto may be served as a dip, on our Svelte Pizzas (see recipe on page 168–170), in our Lotus Liz"agna" (see recipe on page 204), drizzled on salads, as a marinade for tofu, or as a spread on sandwiches. Serves 6–8.

  ½ cup raw pecans
  Himalayan salt coarsely ground (to taste)
  2 cups packed basil leaves
  ⅓ cup olive oil
  3 medium garlic cloves
  ½ cup grated Parmesan (optional)

1. Toast nuts in a medium skillet over low-medium heat, adding salt to taste throughout the process, until golden brown and fragrant. Remove from heat.
2. Place toasted pecans and remaining ingredients in a food processor and pulse until well combined. Serve.

BREATH

"Breath is the bridge which connects life to consciousness, which unites your body to your thoughts."
THICH NHAT HANH

Yoga teaches us to look inward and focus on the breath, *pranayama*. Through steady, elongated, and controlled breathing, we find a stillness of being and a deeper sense of awareness. By focusing on steady breathing during our meals we learn to savor our food experiences. This awareness may also help us to discover when we are hungry and when we are satiated.

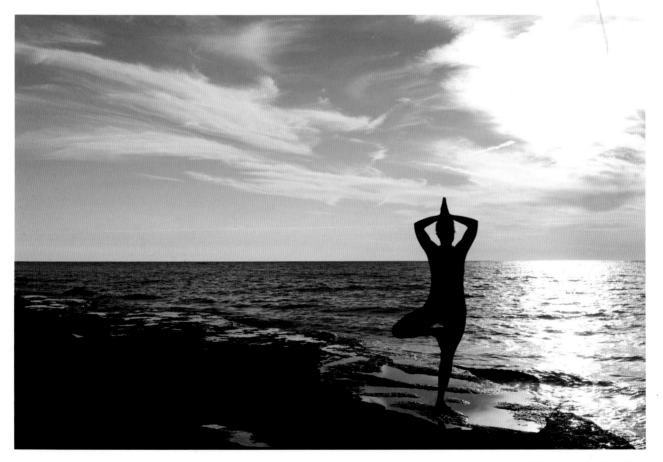

Vrksasana I • Tree Pose

PRESENCE

"Silence is not an absence. Silence is a presence."
LIZ PRICE-KELLOGG

Life is so much more beautiful through the eyes of an observer than through the lens of a smart phone or tablet. When you are practicing yoga, practice yoga. When you are making dinner, make dinner; smell it, feel it, taste it. Engage all of your senses. When you are sitting on the couch, sit on the couch. When you are driving, drive (for your safety and the safety of others). Revel in the presence of even the most seemingly mundane moments.

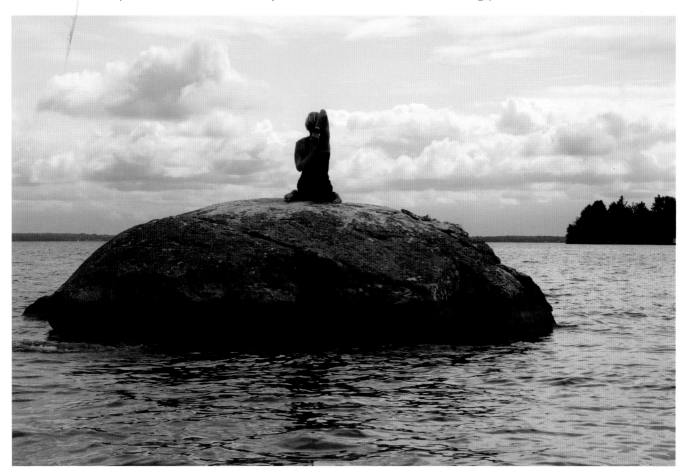

Virasana • Hero Pose

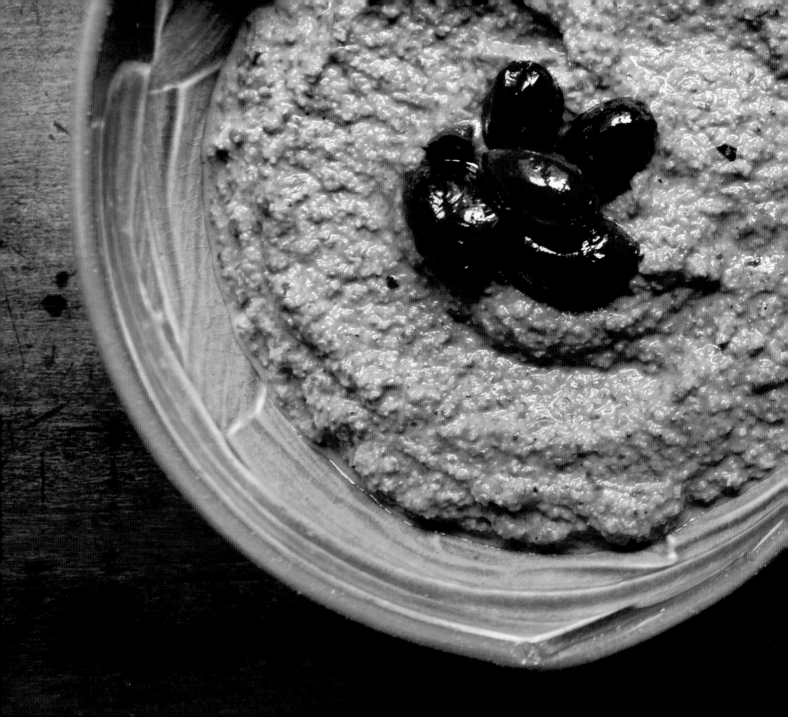

WONDROUS WALNUT & ROASTED RED PEPPER DIP *(v)*

We love foods that originate from the Middle East, India, and Asia, as they are often so wondrous in flavor. This dip was described as "better than hummus" by Liz's husband, Jeremy. It is derived from a classic Middle Eastern dip called Muhammara, but ours uses a fig fruit paste instead of pomegranate molasses (which is traditionally used in this dish, but may not be readily available everywhere and to everyone). Serve the dip with fresh veggies or toasted pita points. It may also be used as a spread on sandwiches or as a base for pizzas! Makes about 3 cups of dip. Serves 8–10.

1 cup raw walnuts
Himalayan salt coarsely ground (to taste)
1 cup roasted red peppers from jar (drained)
¼ cup breadcrumbs
½ cup yellow onion (cut into large pieces)
4–5 medium garlic cloves
3T lemon juice
2T fig fruit paste
1 tsp. cumin
1 tsp. red pepper flakes
1 tsp. paprika
3T olive oil

¼ cup Kalamata olives for garnish (optional)

Pita points (oven toasted and brushed with olive oil) for serving

1. Toast nuts in a medium skillet over low-medium heat, adding salt to taste throughout the process, until golden brown and fragrant.
2. Combine toasted walnuts and remaining ingredients (excluding olives and pita points) in food processor. Pulse until mixture reaches a uniform consistency.
3. Pour dip into a serving bowl. Top with olives and serve with toasted pita points.

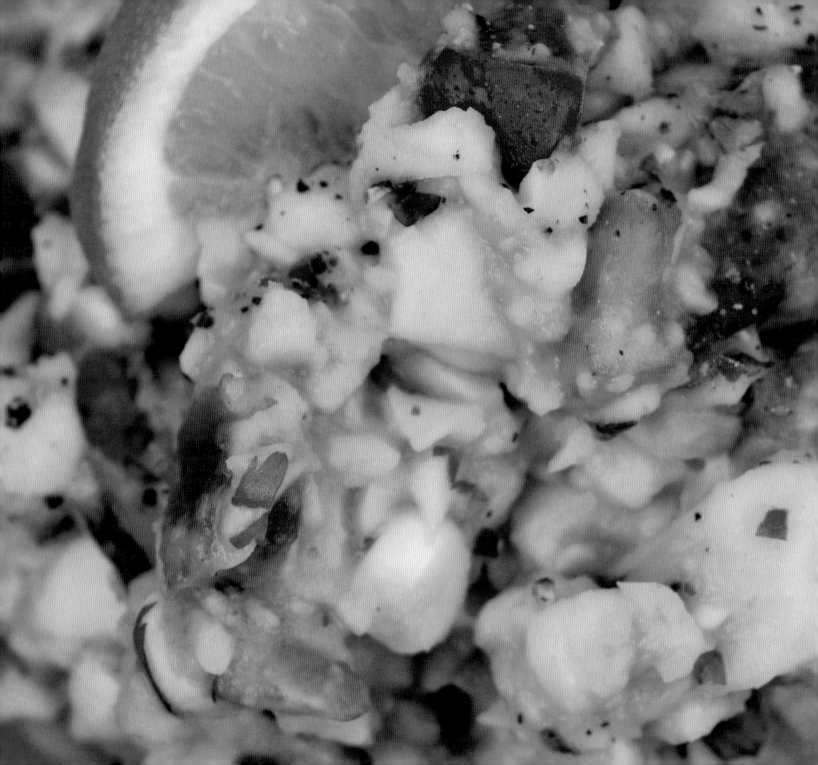

HOLY GUACAMOLE *(v)(r)*

Holy moly, this guacamole is delicious and nutritious! Avocados have been shown to lower cholesterol levels, promote eye health, and protect against cancer. Our Holy Guacamole may be stored in the refrigerator for up to three days. Place plastic wrap directly on top of guacamole if storing in the refrigerator to prevent dip from browning. Serves 8–10.

4 ripe avocados
¼ cup red onion (minced)
1 jalapeño (seeded, de-ribbed, and minced)
4 dashes chipotle hot sauce (optional)
1 small tomato (finely diced)
½ cup cilantro (roughly chopped)
4T lime juice
2 medium garlic cloves (pressed)
½ cup fresh sweet corn
Himalayan salt coarsely ground (to taste)
Pepper coarsely ground (to taste)

1. Cut avocados in half, remove pits, and place fruit of avocados in a medium mixing bowl. Roughly mash avocados with the back of a spoon or potato masher.
2. Place remaining ingredients in bowl and combine.
3. Serve with nutritious chips or vegetables.

BE

The stillness we seek
comes from within.

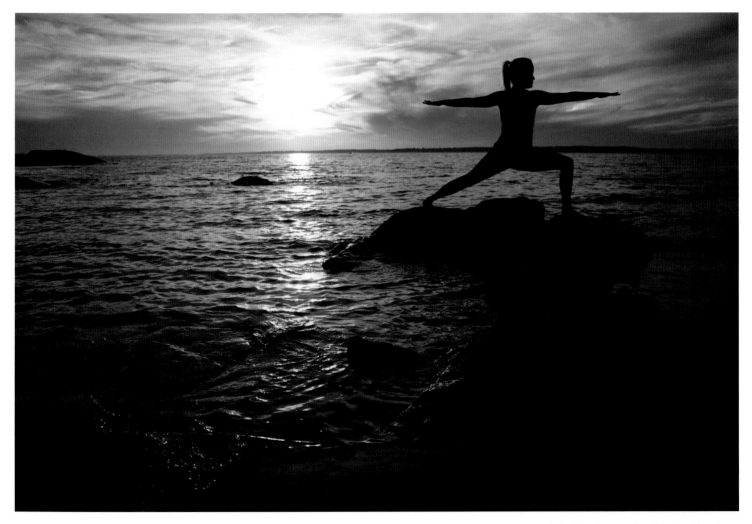

Virabhadrasana II • Warrior Pose Two

HAPPY

"Sometimes your joy is the source of your smile, but sometimes your smile can be the source of your joy."
THICH NHAT HANH

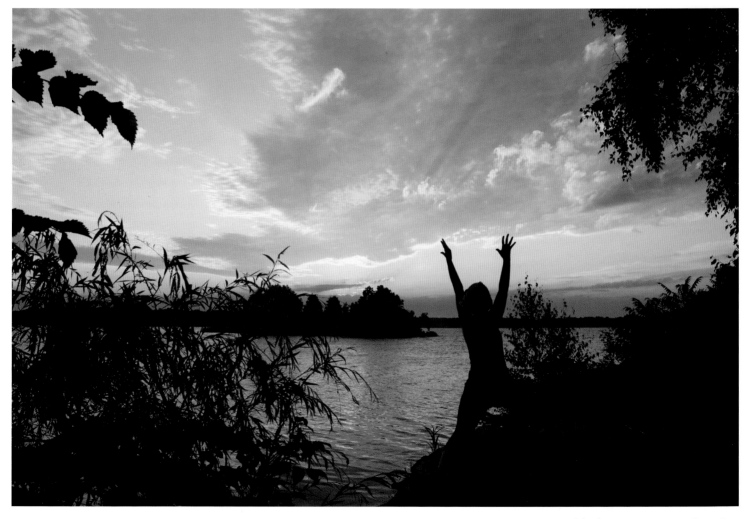

Virabhadrasana I • Warrior Pose One

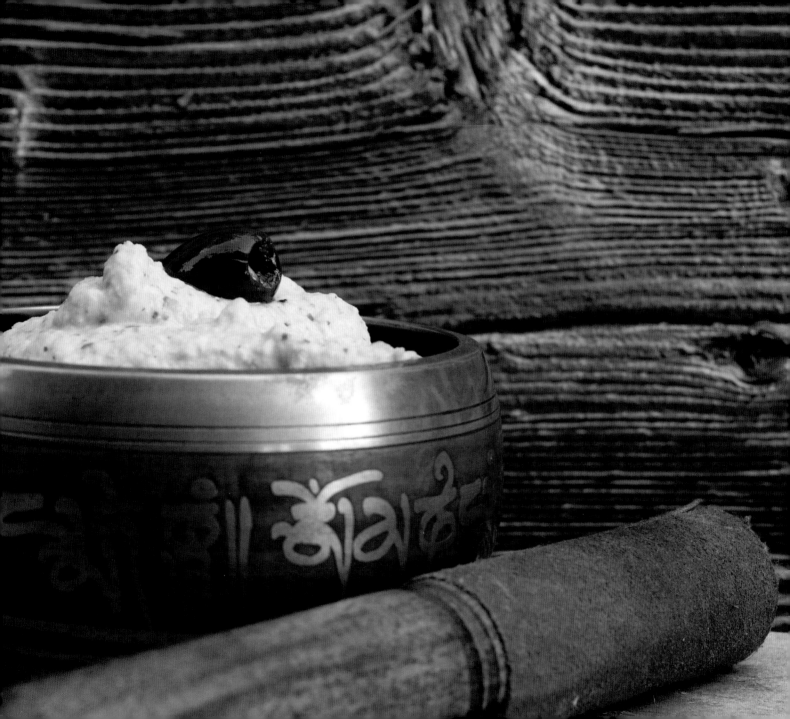

BABA GANESH *(v)*

This is a variation of a classic Middle Eastern dip, Baba Ganoush, which boasts a smoked flavor from charred eggplant. Eggplant may promote cardiovascular health and is packed with vitamins and minerals. The name for this recipe was derived from the name of a Hindu deity, Ganesha. This deity is often depicted with an elephant head, making him easy to identify, and is widely thought of as the remover of obstacles and for his intellect and wisdom. Serves 8–10.

2 large eggplants
½ cup tahini
5 medium garlic cloves (minced)
⅓ cup fresh lemon juice (plus more as needed)
Dash of cumin
Himalayan salt coarsely ground (to taste)
Pepper coarsely ground (to taste)
2T olive oil (plus more for garnish)
2T chopped fresh flat-leaf parsley (plus more for garnish)

1/4 cup Kalamata olives

1. Preheat oven to 400°F.
2. Pierce skin of eggplants with a fork in several places. Evenly char outside of whole eggplants directly on a gas stove flame or under a broiler.
3. Place charred eggplants on a baking sheet and roast until fork tender or for about 30 minutes. Remove from oven and let cool.
4. Scrape out insides of eggplants with a spoon. Place eggplant (without skins) into food processor and blend with remaining ingredients (excluding olives).
5. Pour mixture into a bowl and garnish dip with chopped parsley, olives, and a drizzle of olive oil.

DEDICATIONS

Before each meal and yoga practice, we may choose to offer a personal dedication or prayer. Dedications may be religious, spiritual, simply from the heart, or may stem from another belief system. They may be a showing of thankfulness for all the hands that brought food to the table or even for life's challenges and opportunities. Ultimately, dedications help to make a connection between the meals we are eating, the practices we are experiencing, the people with whom we may be celebrating, the moments that shape our experiences, or possibly, a universal vibration.

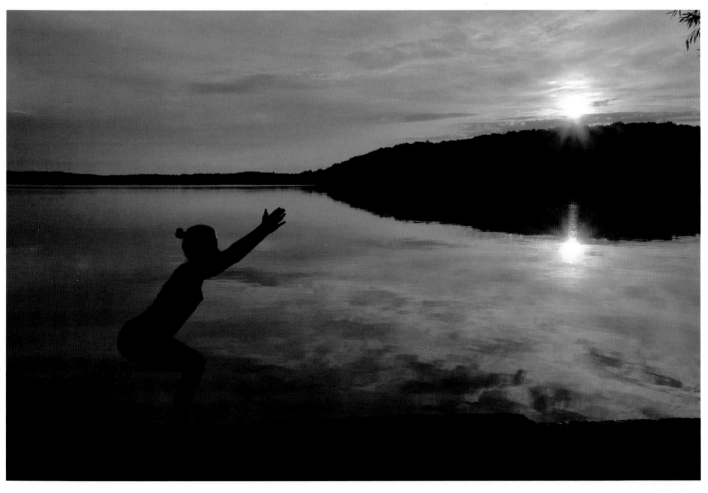

Utkatasana • Chair Pose

ABUNDANCE

"Gratitude is the door to abundance."
YOGI BHAJAN

Don't count your calories.
Count your blessings.

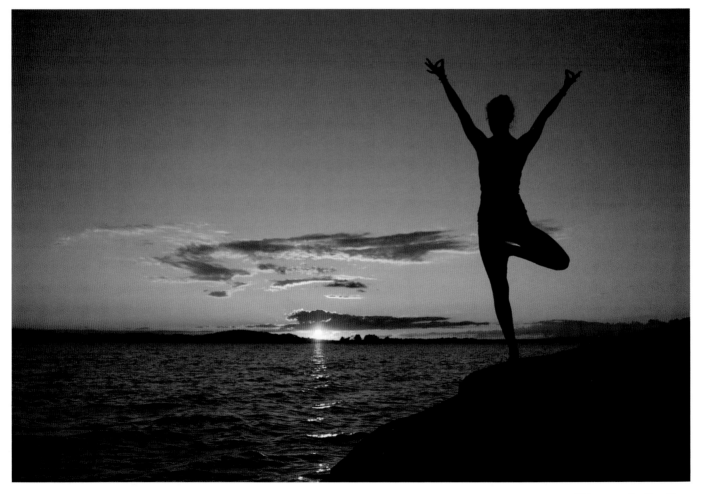

Vrksasana I • Tree Pose

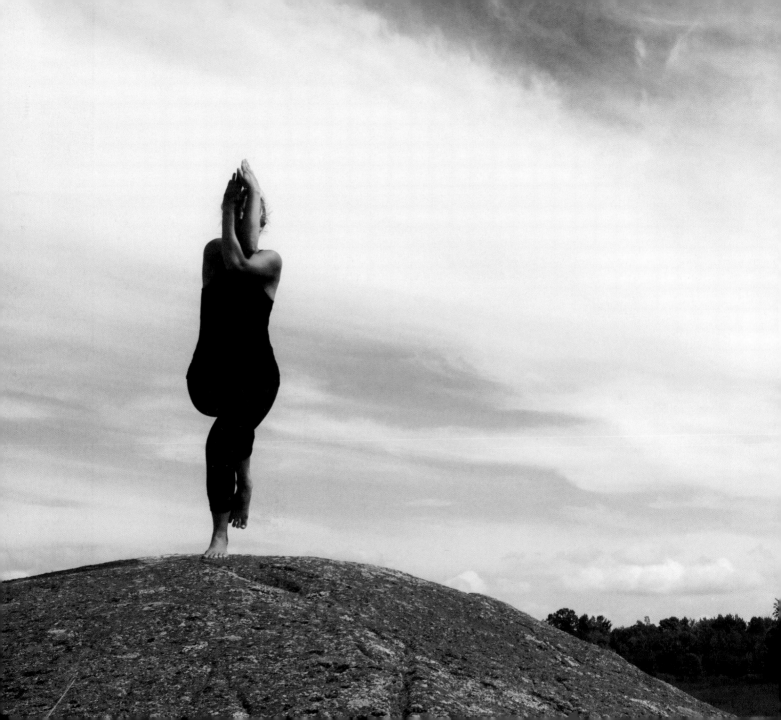

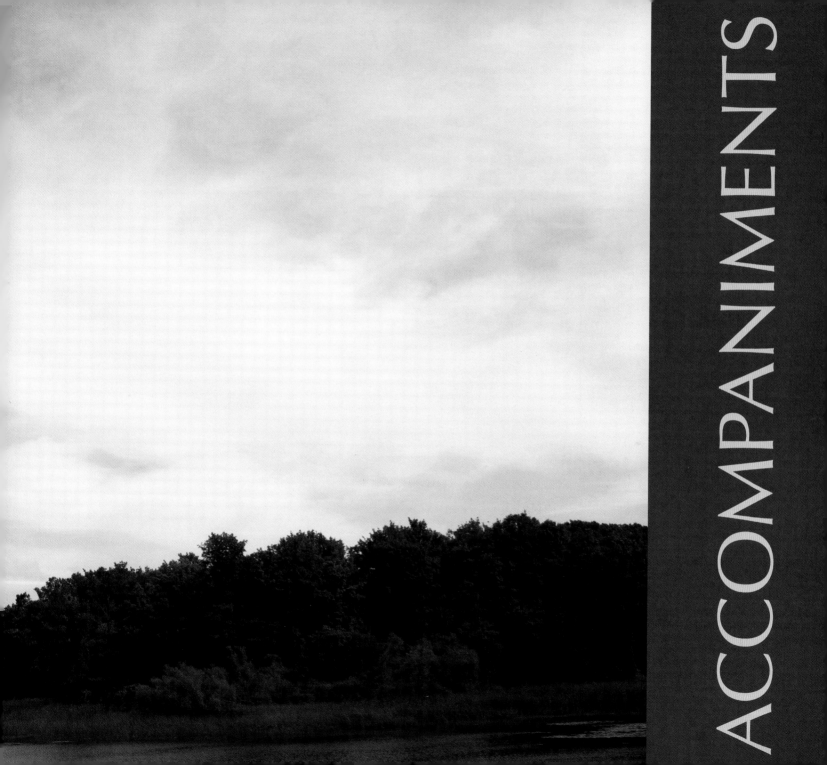

ACCOMPANIMENTS

COMMON SENSE

"You are what you eat."
ANTHELME BRILLAT-SAVARIN

When we utilize our senses of sound, sight, smell, taste, touch, humor, space, time, and spirit, we are using common sense. In our yoga practices, that may mean feeling and listening to the pace of our breath. Our bodies may be telling us to modify or dig deeper into our postures. When we eat, the tastes and smells of our foods may be telling us what and how much to eat. Our modern environments often overshadow common sense. Listen to what makes "common sense" to you.

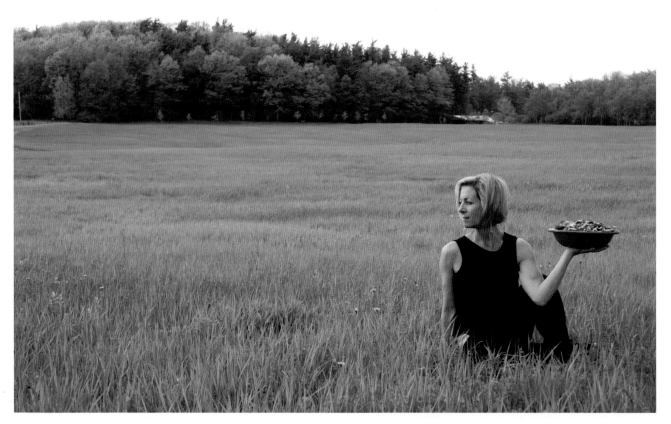

Ardha Matsyendrasana • Half Lord of the Fishes Pose

MEDICINE CABINET

"Let food be thy medicine and medicine be thy food."
HIPPOCRATES

Ancient and modern medicine research concur that one of the best ways to fight illness, prevent disease, heal the body, and incorporate vitamins and minerals into our diets is through eating a variety of healthy, wholesome foods. Herbs and spices featured in our recipes, including basil, capsaicin spices, cinnamon, coriander, garlic, ginger, lavender, oregano, tarragon, and thyme, provide nutritional and wellness benefits and add layered tastes to the foods we share and love.

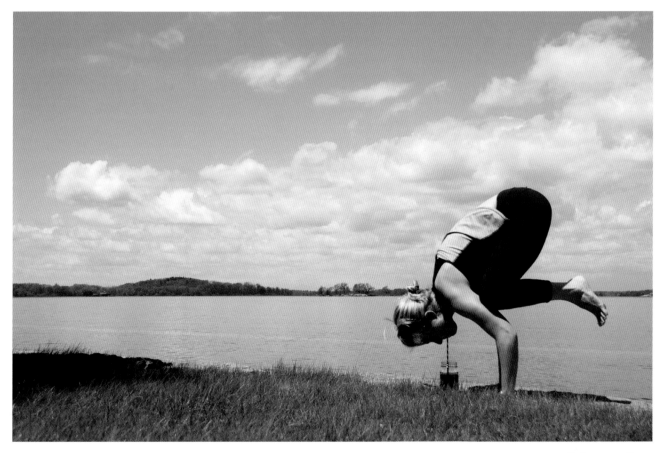

Bakasana • Crow

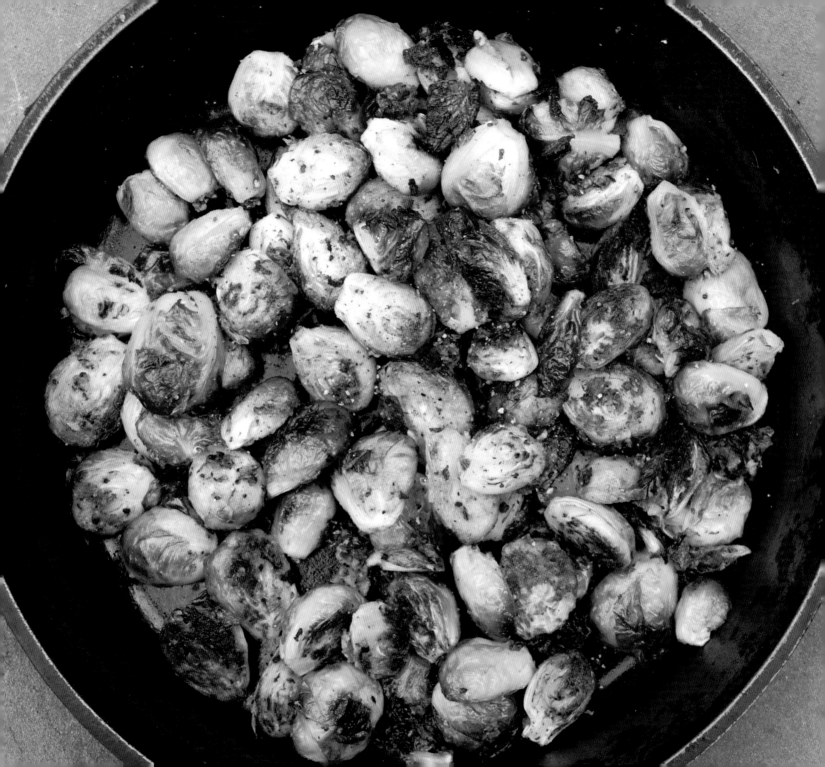

BUDDHA BRUSSELS (v)

"A recipe has no soul. You, as the cook, must bring soul to the recipe."
THOMAS KELLER

Gautama Buddha was a sage and founder of Buddhism, a religion that, among other teachings, embraces the importance of awareness and mindfulness.

Our oven-roasted Brussels sprouts recipe was mindfully created with love. Brussels sprouts provide a variety of health benefits, including lowering cholesterol and protecting our DNA. Get ready to taste, smile, and feel a bit more enlightened. Serves 4–6.

> 20–30 medium Brussels sprouts
> 3 medium garlic cloves (pressed)
> 4T olive oil
> 2T (heaping) Dijon mustard
> Dash of cayenne pepper
> Himalayan salt coarsely ground (to taste)
> Pepper coarsely ground (to taste)

1. Preheat oven to 375°F.
2. Trim, rinse, dry and halve Brussels sprouts.
3. Mix Brussels sprouts with remaining ingredients in bag or bowl and combine well.
4. Place mixture on lightly greased baking sheet and shake ingredients into flat layer.
5. Place in oven and roast for 30 minutes or until outer layers of Brussels sprouts begin to caramelize or crisp.
6. Serve immediately and savor!

SILENCE

"Before you speak, ask yourself, is it kind, is it necessary, is it true, does it improve on the silence?"
SAI BABA

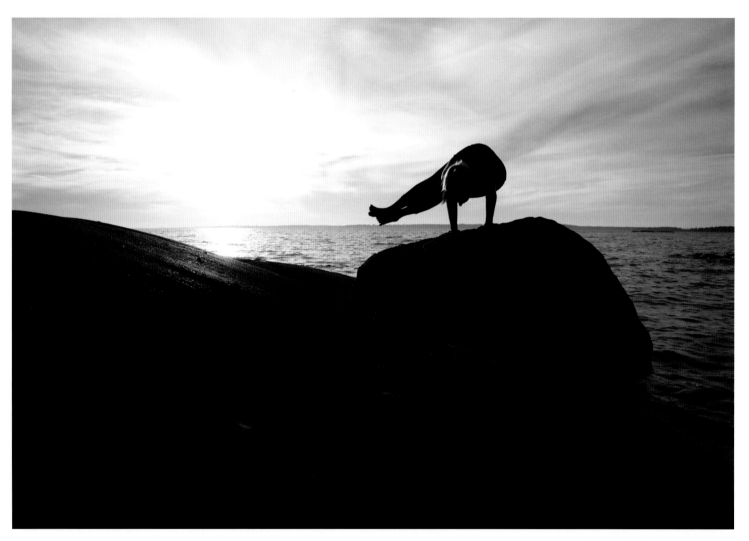

Parsva Bakasana • Side Crow

WISDOM

"Yoga has also been described as wisdom in work or skillful living amongst activities, harmony, and moderation."
B.K.S. IYENGAR

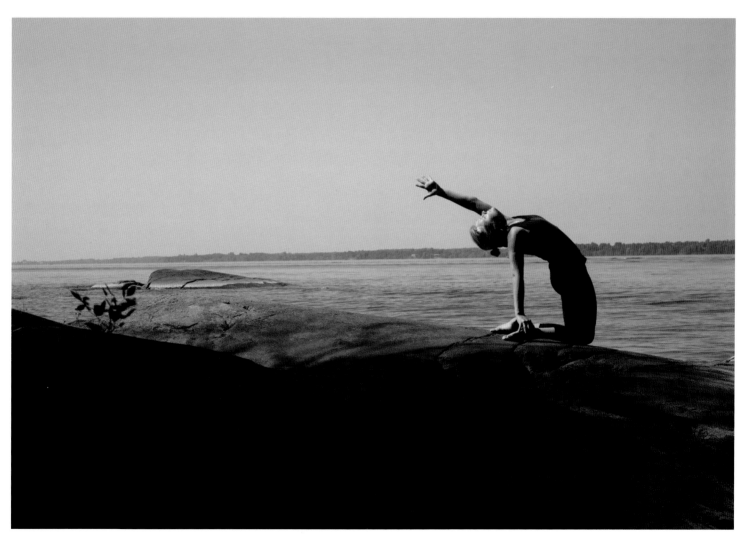

Ardha Ustrasana • Half Camel Posture

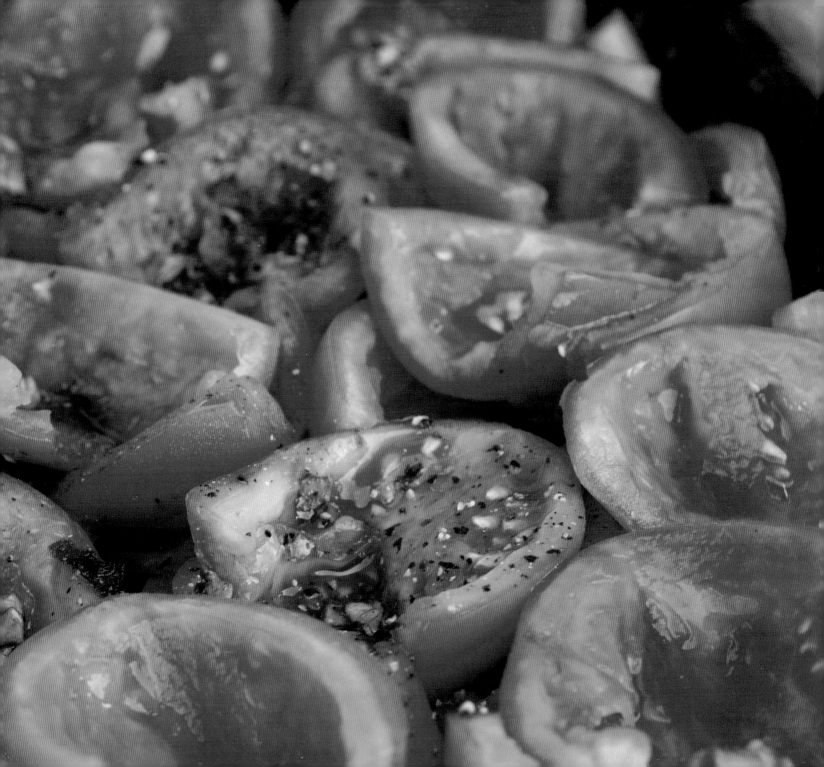

REALIZED ROASTED TOMATOES (v)

Once roasted, these tomatoes boast a wonderfully robust flavor and can be used with a variety of dishes—as tomatoes for our Tantalizing Toasted Herb Svelte Pizza (see recipe on page 168) or in our Humble Hero Greek-style salad (see recipe on page 130)—or served simply as they are as an appetizer or side for an entrée. As a bonus beyond great taste, the nutrients in tomatoes help to promote healthy skin and bones. Tomatoes also contain lycopene, which may greatly reduce the risk of developing certain cancers. Serves 8–10.

    15 plum tomatoes
    5T olive oil
    3T balsamic vinegar
    4 medium garlic cloves (minced)
    2T agave nectar
    Himalayan salt coarsely ground (to taste)
    Pepper coarsely ground (to taste)
    1T fresh oregano (chopped)

1. Preheat oven to 400°F.
2. Cut plum tomatoes lengthwise. Remove cores and seeds.
3. Combine oil, vinegar, garlic, agave, salt, pepper, and oregano to make dressing.
4. Place tomatoes cored side up on a parchment-lined baking sheet. Drizzle oil mixture over tomatoes evenly.
5. Roast for about 30 minutes to 1 hour, or until tomatoes begin to shrink in size, brown, and caramelize.

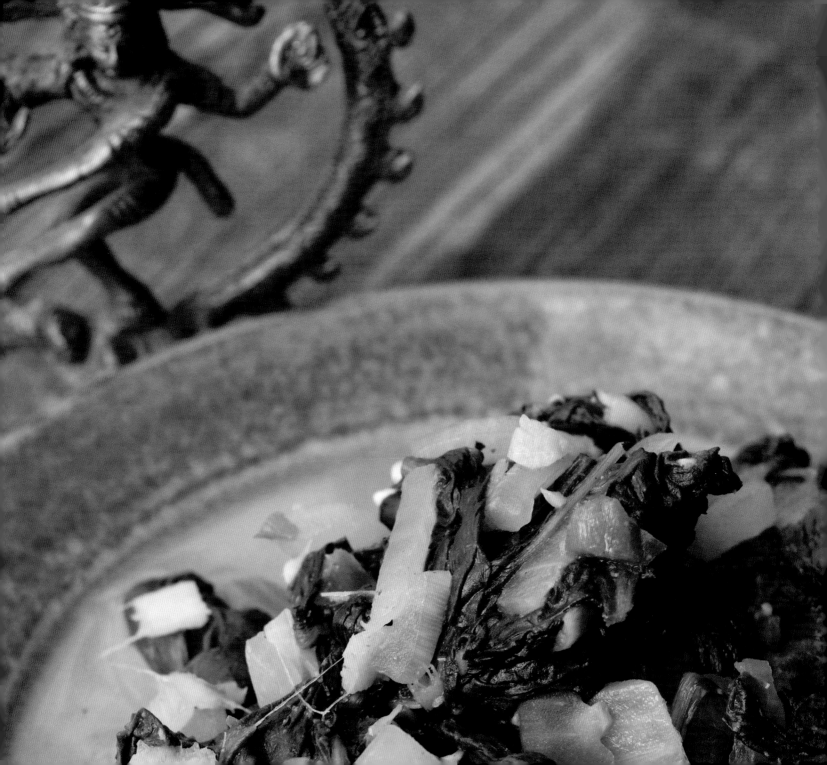

SHIVA SPINACH & CHEESE

A Hindu deity, Shiva is known as the "destroyer of illusion" or the destroyer of ego. When we do not allow our egos to guide our thoughts and actions, our truths are unveiled. In our yoga practices, we sometimes use the hand position Shiva Linga Mudra, which may help to restore confidence and relieve tension.

Our Shiva Spinach & Cheese is a variation of the classic Indian dish—Saag Paneer. This recipe uses feta instead of paneer, the Indian cheese classically used in this dish. Variation: If you are able to easily find paneer, it may be used instead of the feta. Eating iron-rich spinach may aid in diabetes management as well as cancer and asthma prevention. The dish also incorporates a variety of spices that we love for their healing and nutritional benefits. Cayenne pepper and cumin contain capsaicin, are an anti-inflammatory and have anti-cancer properties. Serves 4–8.

¼ tsp. turmeric
Dash of cayenne pepper (to taste)
Himalayan salt coarsely ground (to taste)
Pepper coarsely ground (to taste)
¼ cup crumbled feta cheese
1T olive oil
1 large white onion (minced)
1½T fresh ginger (minced)
4 large garlic cloves (minced)
1 Serrano chili (seeded, de-ribbed, and minced)
½ tsp. ground garam masala
1 tsp. ground coriander
1 tsp. ground cumin
8 cups fresh baby spinach leaves (coarsely chopped)
¾ cup vegetable broth

1. Combine turmeric, cayenne, salt, and pepper in a medium mixing bowl. Add feta and combine. Set aside.
2. In a large skillet over low-medium heat, add olive oil, onion, ginger, garlic, and chili. Sauté ingredients for about 10 minutes. Add the garam masala, coriander, and cumin. Sauté for another minute.
3. Add the chopped spinach and combine with the other ingredients until mostly wilted or for about 5 minutes. Add vegetable broth to the mixture and bring to a simmer, uncovered, for about 5 minutes or until broth is mostly absorbed.
4. Remove the mixture from heat and add feta. Combine. Allow the dish to rest for about 3–5 minutes to allow the flavors to marry. Serve and enjoy.

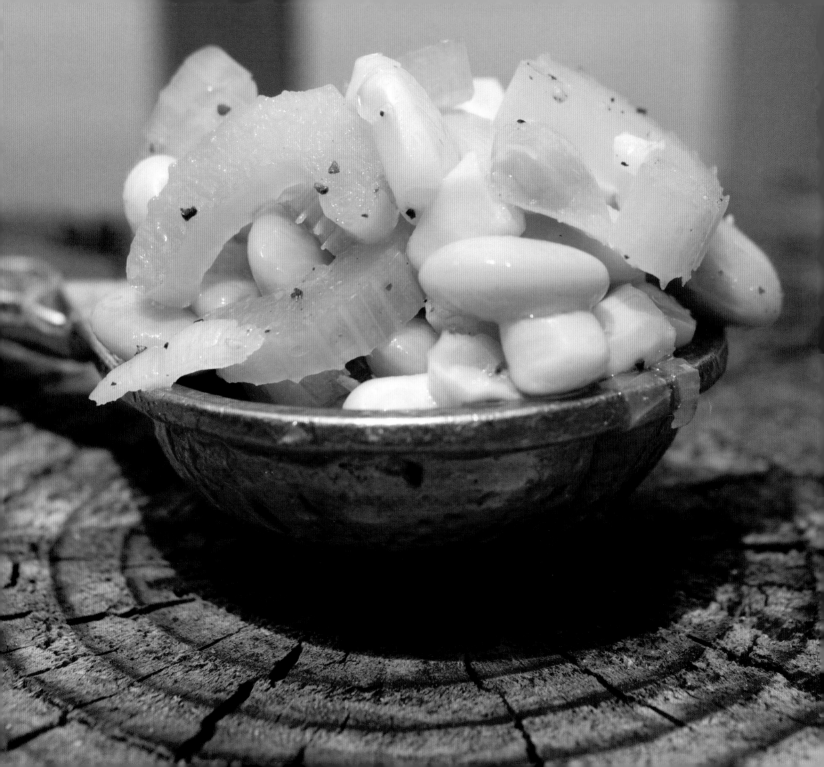

BALANCED BUTTER BEANS (v)

Yoga is an inward journey where our steady breath helps us to find balance. As the name of this recipe implies, the ingredients are perfectly balanced, creating a blissful dining experience. "Butter beans" are actually just large lima beans. While we always recommend buying fresh ingredients, flash frozen organic lima beans also work well for this dish. The lemon and agave dressing for this dish is light and delicious. The inclusion of celery provides a great crunch. Serves 10–12. (This dish may be made a day ahead of time and stored in the refrigerator for up to a week.)

2 lbs. lima beans
1½ cups corn kernels (cut fresh off of the cob)
1 cup celery (chopped)
½ cup scallions (chopped)
¾ cups lemon juice
¼ cup cider vinegar
3T agave nectar
1 large shallot (minced)
¾ cup olive oil
Himalayan salt coarsely ground (to taste)
Pepper coarsely ground (to taste)

1. Combine lima beans, corn, celery, and scallions in a large bowl.
2. Combine lemon juice, vinegar, agave, shallot, olive oil, salt, and pepper to taste to make dressing.
3. Pour dressing over salad and combine. Serve at room temperature.

VRKSASANA I
TREE POSE

balancing, strengthening, helps to focus the mind

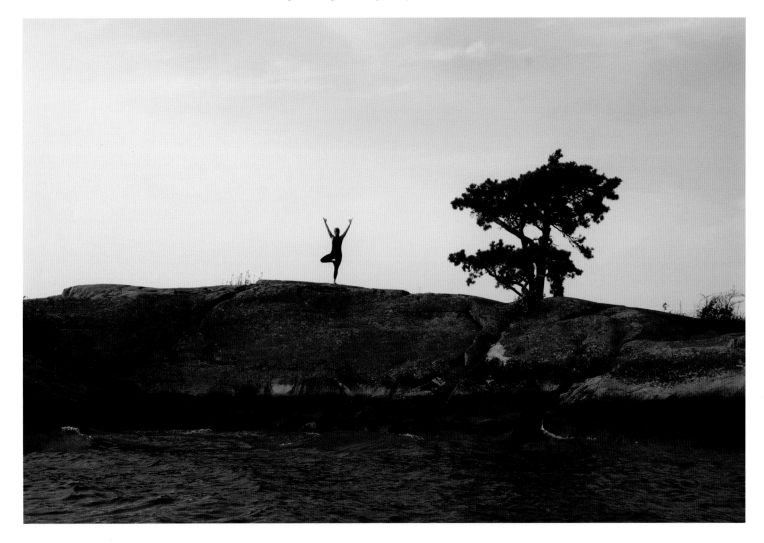

BALANCE

THE PARADOX OF OUR AGE

We have bigger houses but smaller families;
more conveniences, but less time;
We have more degrees, but less sense;
more knowledge, but less judgment;
more experts, but more problems;
more medicines, but less healthiness;
We've been all the way to the moon and back,
but have trouble crossing the street to meet
the new neighbor.
We've built more computers to hold more
information to produce more copies than ever,
but have less communications;
We have become long on quantity,
but short on quality.
These times are times of fast foods;
but slow digestion;
Tall man but short character;
Steep profits but shallow relationships.
It is time when there is much in the window,
but nothing in the room.

HIS HOLINESS THE XIV DALAI LAMA

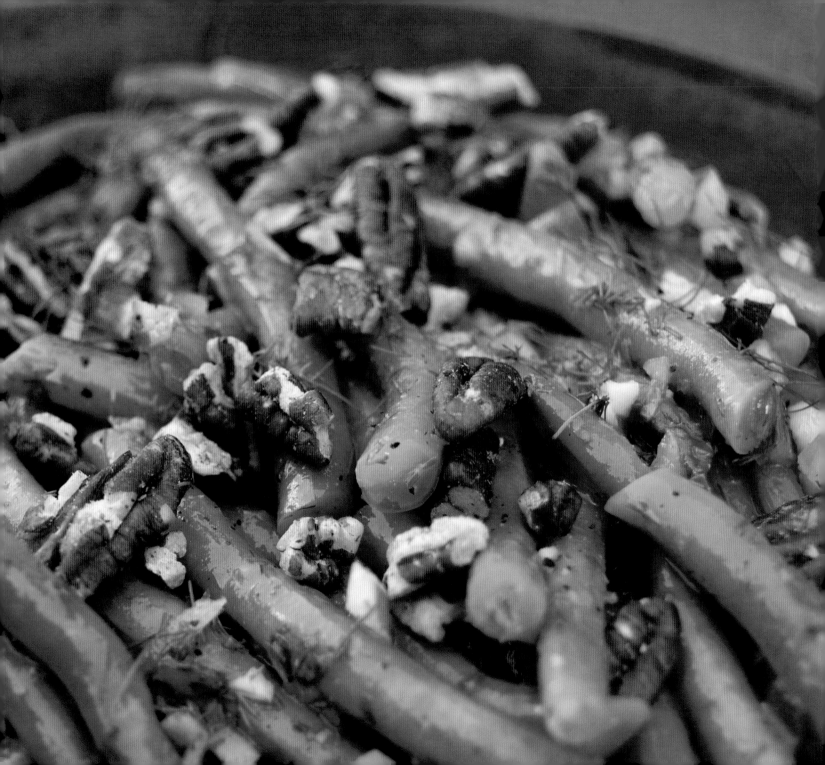

OM MY GOODNESS GREEN BEANS *(v)*

Om, which is written as "aum" in Sanskrit, is a sound or mantra that connects us to universal consciousness. Though these green beans may not have a divine energy, we believe they have great energy and are delicious. The citrus notes derived from the fresh orange juice and the white wine vinegar enliven the dish and serve as a refreshing complement to the strong dill, garlic, and red onion flavors. Thank you to our friend, Sheri, for inspiring this dish. You remind us to "let all of the flavors marry," which is the last step of this recipe. Our Simply Perfect Pecans top this dish. Serves 4–6.

2 lbs. fresh green beans (trimmed and rinsed)

⅓ cup pecans

¾ cup olive oil
½ cup white wine vinegar
1T Dijon mustard
2T (heaping) orange juice with pulp
3 medium garlic cloves (finely chopped)
⅓ cup red onion (finely chopped)
1 jalapeño (seeded, de-ribbed, and finely chopped)
½ cup fresh basil (chopped)
½ cup dill (chopped)
Himalayan salt coarsely ground (to taste)
Pepper coarsely ground (to taste)

½ cup crumbled feta cheese (optional)

1. In a large saucepan, bring water to a boil. Blanch trimmed and rinsed green beans for 1 minute. Immediately drain and put beans in ice bath or in a bowl in the refrigerator.
2. Toast pecans in cast iron skillet over low-medium heat until golden brown and fragrant. Sprinkle with salt while toasting to taste.
3. Combine remaining ingredients (aside from feta) to make dressing.
4. Combine cool green beans and dressing. Let the flavors marry for at least 30 minutes.
5. Top with feta and toasted pecans before serving. Serve at room temperature.

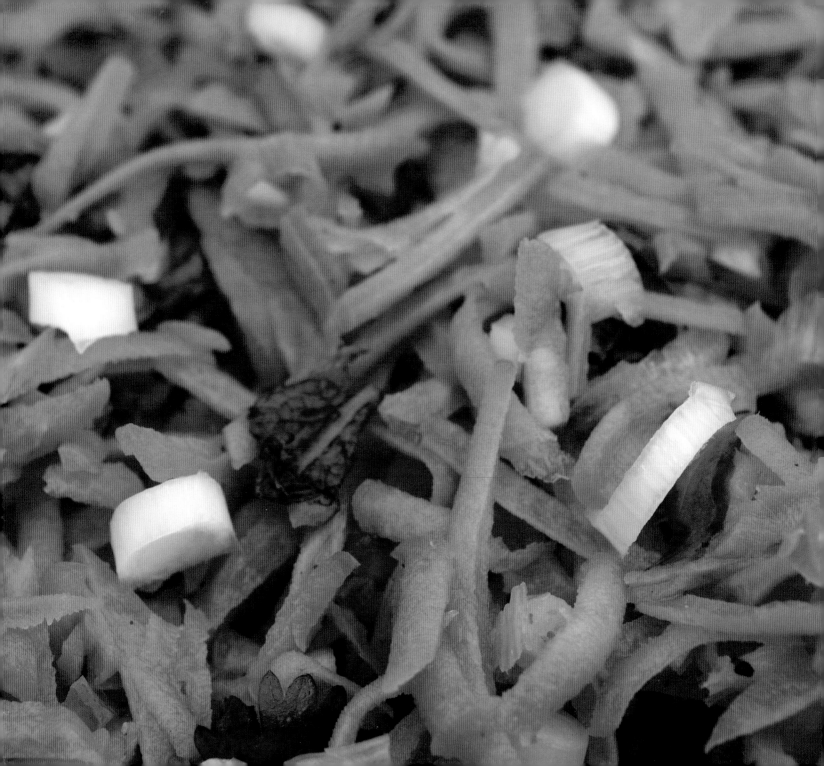

RADIANT CARROTS *(v)(r)*

We love carrots, partially because their nutritional benefits include better eye function and delaying the effects of aging, keeping us feeling young and radiant. The addition of fresh ginger to this salad enlivens the whole dish. Healthy and delicious, this carrot salad may help you glow from the inside out! It is also delicious when added to sandwiches (see our Radiant Carrot Salad Pita recipe on page 180). Serves 8–10.

1 lb. to 1 ½ lbs. carrots, peeled
2T fresh ginger (minced)
1T agave nectar
1 hot pepper (seeded and de-ribbed)
¼ cup red onion (minced)
2 medium garlic cloves (minced)
1T lime juice
3T orange juice
¼ cup mint (chopped)
¼ cup cilantro (chopped)
3T olive oil
Himalayan salt coarsely ground (to taste)
Pepper coarsely ground (to taste)
2T chopped scallions (garnish)

1. Clean and shred carrots.
2. Combine remaining ingredients (except for scallions) in large mixing or serving bowl to make dressing.
3. Combine carrots and dressing and garnish with chopped scallions. Serve at room temperature or cold.

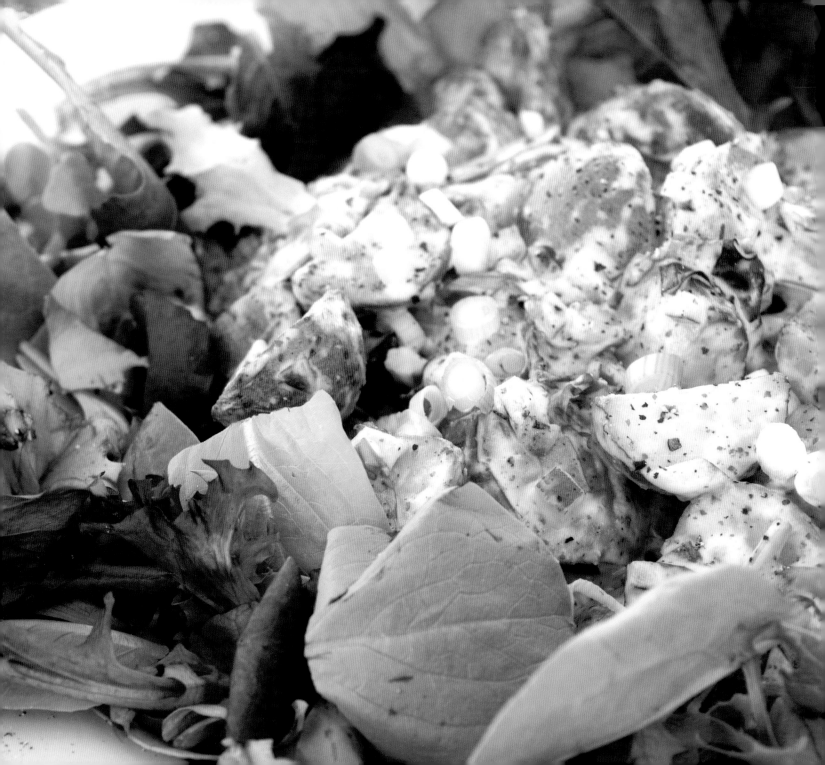

RESTFUL ROSEMARY POTATOES *(v)*

This is probably one of the best good-for-you potato salad recipes you'll find, and we think it is also one of the best-tasting! Rosemary and dark leafy greens add an extra layer of nutrition, texture, and taste to this dish. Serves 4–6.

2 lbs. small multi-colored new potatoes
2T fresh rosemary (chopped)
4 medium garlic cloves (minced)
1T olive oil
Himalayan salt coarsely ground (to taste)
Pepper coarsely ground (to taste)
½ cup vegan mayonnaise
1½T lemon juice
1T Dijon mustard
¼ cup red onion (chopped)
1 cup mixed greens
2T scallions (chopped)

1. Preheat oven to 350°F.
2. Clean potatoes, leaving skins on, and cut them in half lengthwise or quarter into generous bite-sized pieces.
3. Combine potatoes with rosemary, garlic, olive oil, salt, and pepper. Spread onto baking sheet and bake for 45–50 minutes or until potatoes are crisp on the outside, but still slightly al dente inside. Check the potatoes half way through, toss, and season with salt and pepper if needed.
4. Remove potatoes from oven and allow them to rest on the pan until they reach room temperature. (Because they are so delicious, you may choose to eat these potatoes now, but remember they then won't be available for your potato salad.)
5. While potatoes are cooling combine vegan mayonnaise, lemon juice, Dijon, and red onion in a mixing bowl. Set aside until potatoes reach room temperature.
6. Combine cooled potatoes, dressing, and mixed greens. Top with scallions and serve immediately.

UTKATASANA
CHAIR POSE

*even though this sounds relaxing, this pose requires much effort and
is energizing and strengthening*

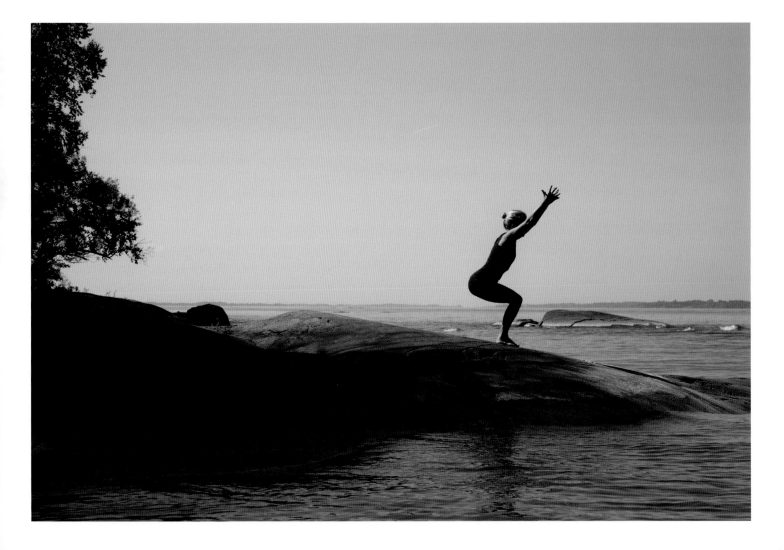

SALAMBA SIRSASANA
SUPPORTED HEADSTAND

liberating, stimulates nervous system, brings clarity, "king of all poses"

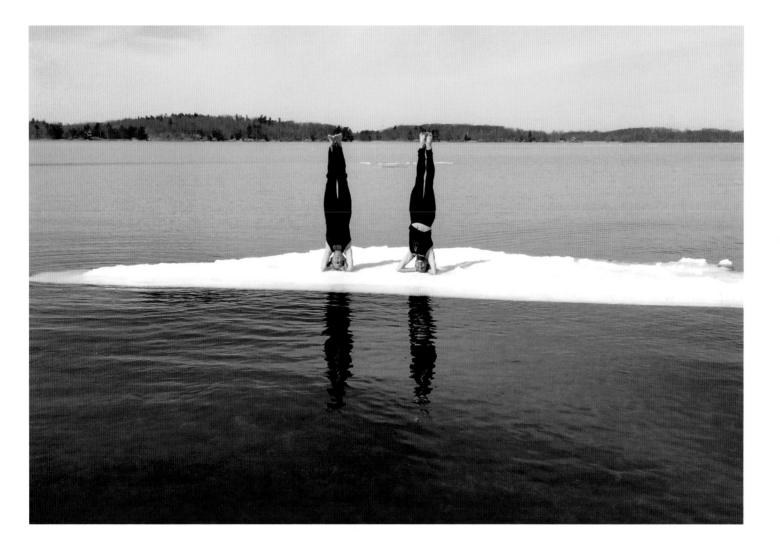

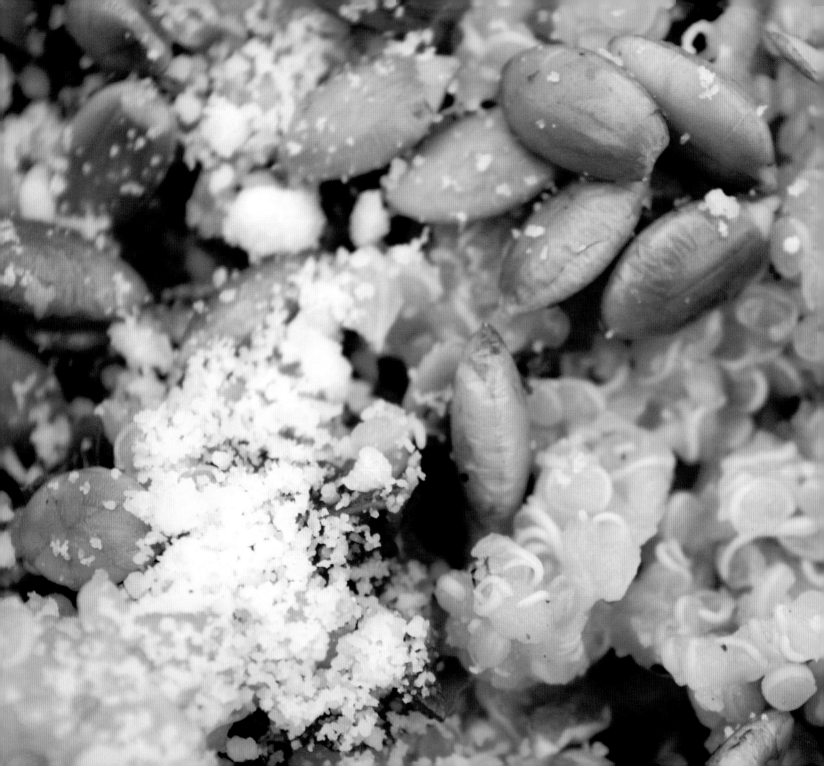

GURU GRAINS *(v)*

In Hinduism and Buddhism a "guru" is a spiritual teacher. Our Guru Grains offer the powers of ancient grains, super greens, and nutrient-rich squash to feed the body and mind. One key to this dish is using a high-quality vegetable broth, whether that originates from stock, bullion cubes, or a concentrated base. Enjoy this quinoa salad at room temperature. It also stores well in the refrigerator and makes for great leftovers. Serves 10–12.

1 large butternut squash (halved)
2T olive oil
½ cup pepitas
½ cup onion (minced)
6 medium garlic cloves (minced)
2 cups kale (cleaned and de-ribbed)
4 cups vegetable broth
2 cups quinoa
Himalayan salt coarsely ground, to taste (plus more for pepitas)
Pepper coarsely ground (to taste)
½ cup freshly grated Parmesan (optional)

1. Preheat oven to 400°F.
2. Bake squash on a baking sheet with 1 tablespoon of olive oil for about 35 minutes or until fork tender. Let the squash rest for about 20 minutes and then remove skin and cut into chunks. Keep warm.
3. Toast pepitas in a skillet over low-medium heat until fragrant and golden brown. Remove from heat and set aside.
4. Sauté onion, garlic, and kale with 1 tablespoon of olive oil in a large skillet over medium heat until kale is slightly softened.
5. Add vegetable broth and quinoa to skillet. Bring to a boil and then reduce temperature to bring mixture to a simmer. Cover and simmer until liquid is absorbed (about 15–30 minutes). Remove from heat and pour off any excess liquid.
6. Stir in squash.
7. Season with additional salt and/or pepper.
8. Top with pepitas and freshly grated Parmesan.

CREATE

"We are not going to change the whole world, but we can change ourselves and feel free as birds. We can be serene even in the midst of calamities and, by our serenity, make others more tranquil . . .

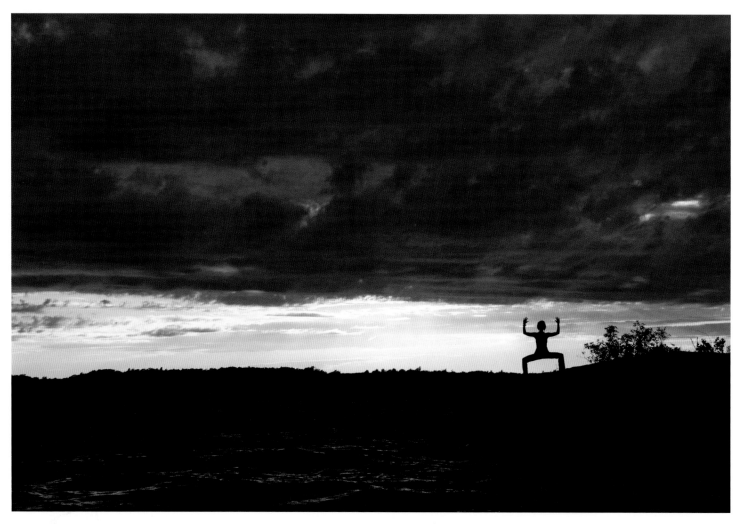

Utkata Konasana • Goddess Pose

JOY

. . . Serenity is contagious. If we smile at someone, he or she will smile back. And a smile costs nothing. We should plague everyone with joy. If we are to die in a minute, why not die happily, laughing?"
SWAMI SATCHIDANANDA, *THE YOGA SUTRAS*

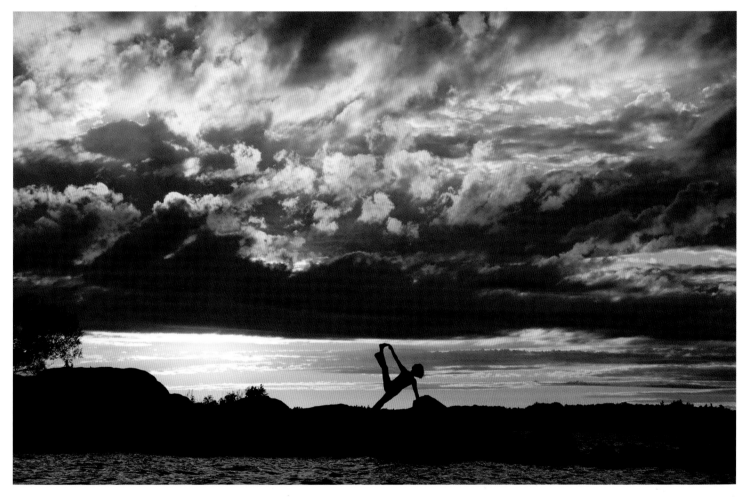

Vasisthasana III • Advanced Side Plank

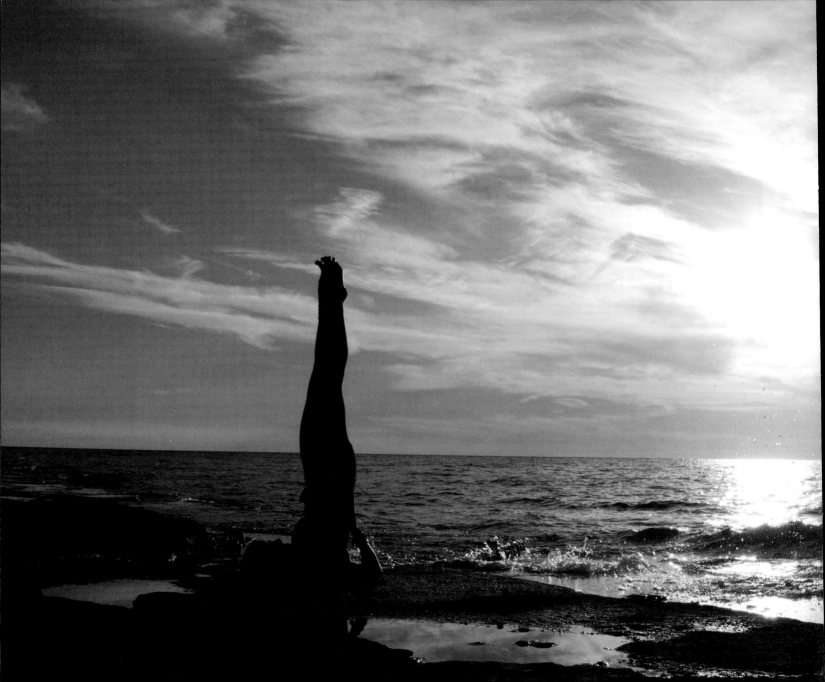

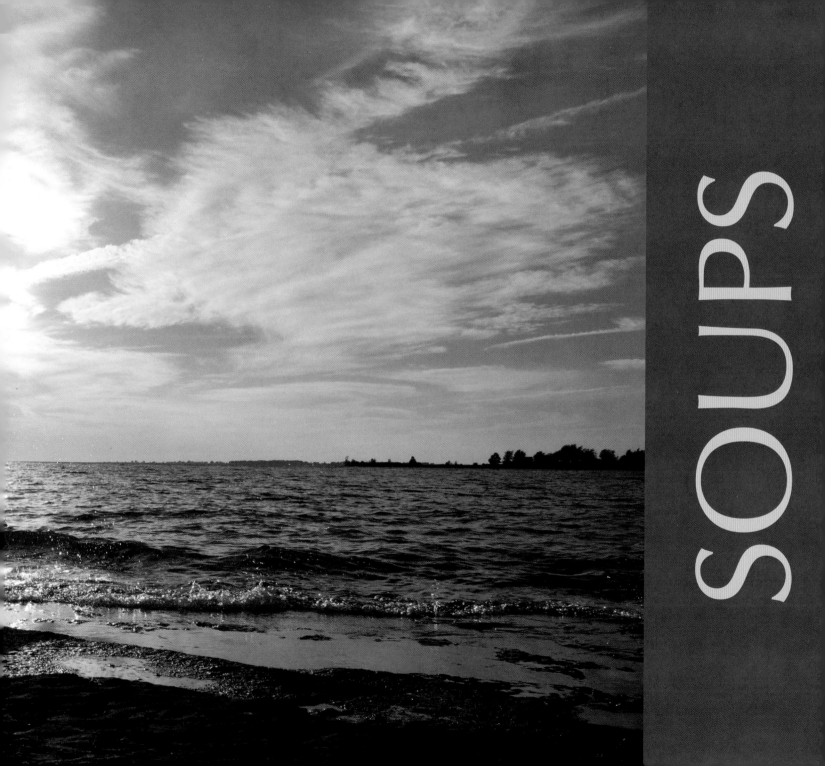

SOUPS

RESPONSIBILITY

"Be the change that you wish to see in the world."
MAHATMA GANDHI

Our yoga practices are moving meditations that offer lessons—non-harming (*ahimsa*), focus, flexibility, gratitude, and contentment—that transcend our mats. As we continue to learn from our yoga practices, we have a responsibility to incorporate these lessons into our daily choices. That in turn will influence and inspire those lives we touch.

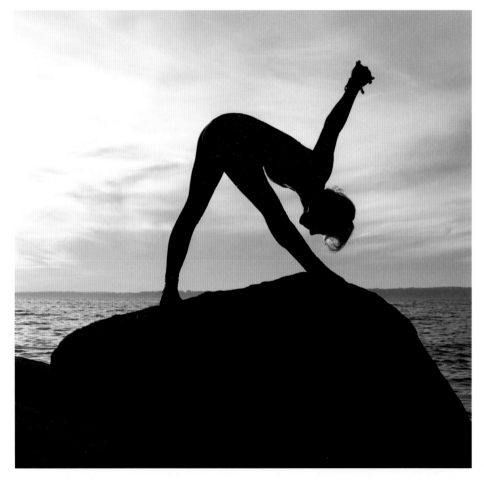

Parsvottanasana • Pyramid Pose

GROWTH

"Watch your thoughts; they become words. Watch your words; they become actions. Watch your actions; they become habits. Watch your habits; they become character. Watch your character; for it becomes your destiny."
UPANISHADS

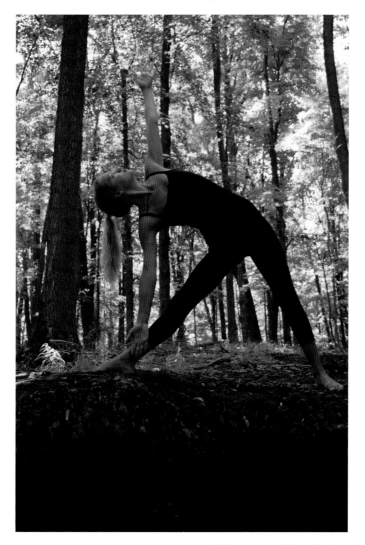

Trikonasana • Triangle Pose

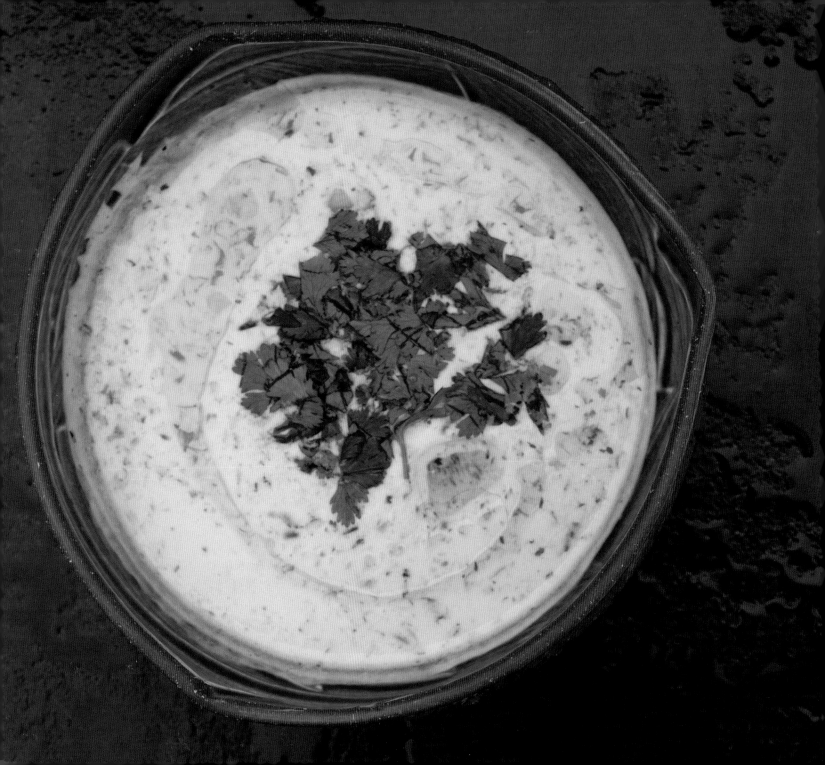

SEDUCTIVE CILANTRO

Coriander and cilantro come from a plant called coriandrum sativum, but they are two different ingredients. Coriander is the seed of the plant, while cilantro is the leaf. Coriander aids in digestion and may help to treat skin inflammation. Cilantro is a powerful herb. It has been shown to act as a cleanser or detoxifier for the body. We fell in love with a version of this cilantro soup at a former neighborhood garden bistro. It is a remarkably soulful, decadent, and even seductive soup, rich with fresh cilantro flavor. Serves 8–10.

    1T olive oil
    4 medium garlic cloves (minced)
    1 white onion (chopped)
    Dash of ground cayenne pepper
    ½ tsp. cumin
    4 cups cilantro (washed and de-stemmed)
    4 cups vegetable broth
    8 oz. cream cheese
    16 oz. sour cream
    Himalayan salt coarsely ground (to taste)
    Pepper coarsely ground (to taste)
    Olive oil (drizzle for garnish)
    Cilantro leaves (garnish)

1. Combine olive oil, garlic, onion, cayenne, and cumin in a large saucepan or Dutch oven over low-medium heat. Cook until vegetables are translucent and softened or for about 5–10 minutes. Set aside.
2. Combine sautéed vegetables with cilantro and 1 cup vegetable broth in food processor. Puree.
3. Transfer ingredients back to the same large saucepan already used. Add remaining broth and bring ingredients to a boil. Stir in cream cheese, sour cream, salt, and pepper. Simmer uncovered for 15 minutes over low heat.
4. Serve in bowls and garnish each bowl with a drizzle of olive oil and cilantro leaves.

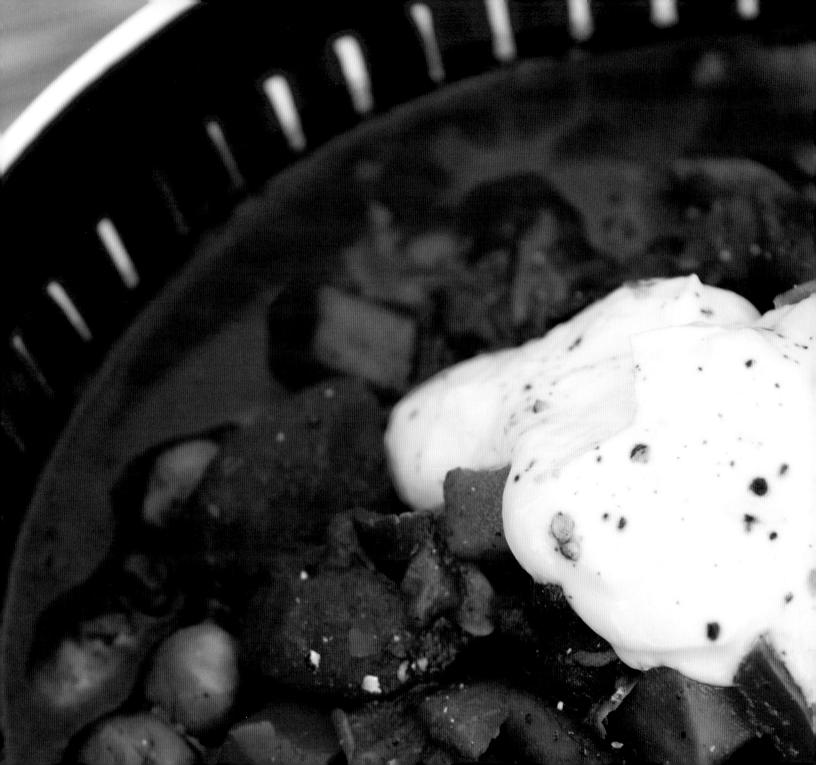

WIND RELEASING CHILI *(v)*

Sing along . . . "Beans, beans, they're good for your heart; the more you eat the more you fart; the more you fart the better you feel; beans, beans for every meal . . ." As the classic song so beautifully implies, beans are packed full of antioxidants and are high in fiber, making them a top-of-the-charts health food. Our vegetarian chili is full of beans and vegetables. It is a hearty and filling soup, and also one that is great to share with family and friends (as long as you feel comfortable singing this song with them . . .). Serves 8.

4T olive oil
1 large white onion (chopped)
1 large carrot (chopped)
2 stalks celery (chopped)
4 medium garlic cloves (minced)
½ Serrano chili pepper (seeded, de-ribbed, and chopped)
2 cups Portobello mushrooms (chopped)
1 red bell pepper (chopped)
1 large zucchini (chopped)
2T cumin
2T chili powder
2T paprika
Dash of cayenne pepper
15 oz. canned kidney beans (drained and rinsed)

15 oz. canned black beans (drained and rinsed)
15 oz. canned chickpeas (drained and rinsed)
1 ½ cups vegetable stock
10–12 medium (diced) or 28 oz. canned chopped tomatoes with juices
Cheesecloth purse (with 2 sprigs of thyme, 2 sprigs of oregano, and 2 bay leaves)
Himalayan salt coarsely ground (to taste)
Pepper coarsely ground (to taste)
1 avocado, sliced (optional, for garnish)
Greek yogurt (strained) or sour cream (optional, for garnish)
Green onions, chopped (optional, for garnish)
Grated cheese (optional, for garnish)

1. In a large saucepan or Dutch oven over medium heat, sauté onion, carrot, celery, garlic, chili peppers, mushrooms, red bell pepper, and zucchini in olive oil until translucent and softened or about 5–10 minutes.
2. Add remaining ingredients (excluding garnishes) to saucepan and bring to a boil. Reduce heat to low and simmer ingredients for about 45 minutes to 1 hour. Season to taste with salt and pepper.
3. Remove cheesecloth purse.
4. Place in individual bowls and top with optional garnishes as desired.

URDHVA PAVANAMUKTASANA
STANDING WIND RELIEVING OR KNEE-TO-CHEST POSE

excellent for relieving abdominal gas!

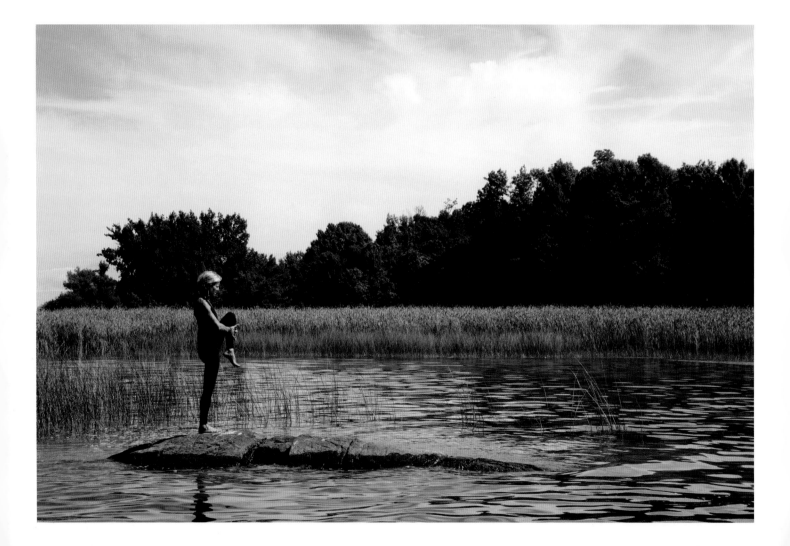

VRSCHIKASANA
SCORPION

strengthens, invigorates

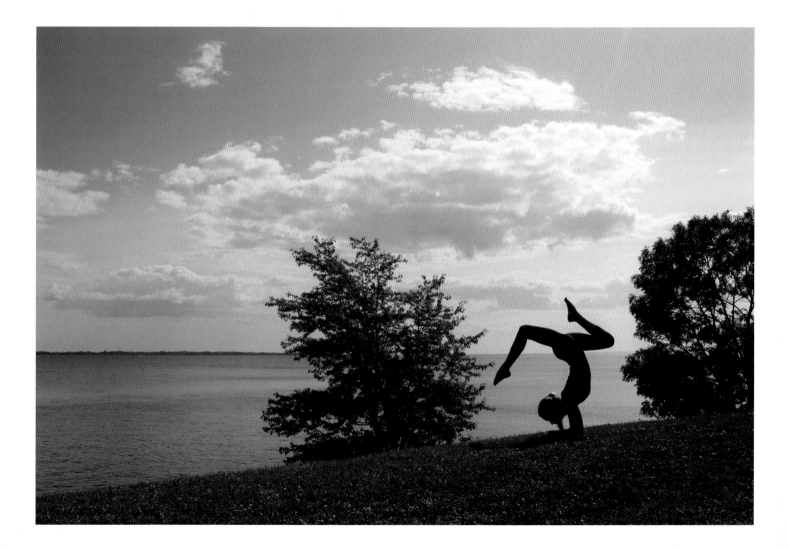

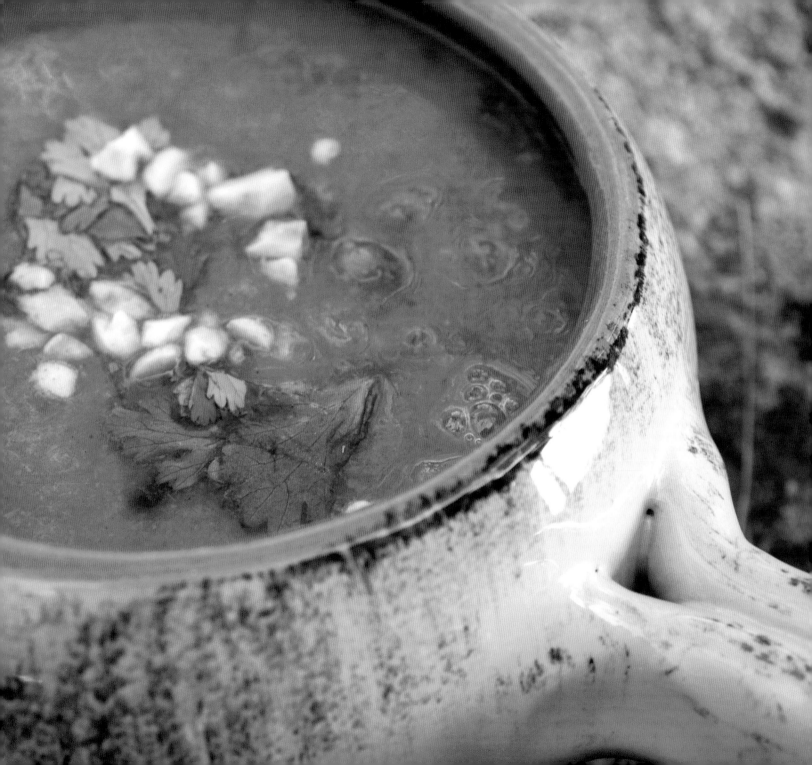

SCORPION SWEET POTATO *(v)*

We are excited to include this South African–inspired soup in our catalog of recipes. Sweet potatoes, also called yams, are bursting with antioxidants and may help to balance the body's hormonal levels. They are also full of fiber and naturally sweet, which helps to regulate blood sugar levels and reduce fatigue. Serves 8–10.

2T olive oil
2T fresh ginger (chopped)
4 medium garlic cloves (chopped)
1 yellow onion (chopped)
1 red bell pepper (chopped)
½ Serrano pepper (seeded, de-ribbed, and chopped)
¼ tsp. ground cinnamon
¼ tsp. ground coriander
¼ tsp. ground clove
Dash of cayenne pepper (or to taste)
¼ tsp. cumin
¼ tsp. turmeric
5–6 medium (diced) or 15 oz. chopped tomatoes with juices

2T agave nectar
3 large sweet potatoes (diced)
4 cups vegetable broth
1T red curry paste
Himalayan salt coarsely ground (to taste)
Pepper coarsely ground (to taste)
30 oz. black beans
½ cup chunky peanut butter
½ cup coconut milk
½ cup fresh cilantro leaves (chopped, plus leaves for garnish)
Fresh chopped peanuts (optional for garnish)

1. In a large saucepan or Dutch oven over medium heat, sauté ginger, garlic, onion, bell pepper, and Serrano pepper in olive oil until softened or for about 10 minutes.
2. Add cinnamon, coriander, clove, cayenne, cumin, and turmeric. Continue to sauté for an additional 2–3 minutes.
3. Add tomatoes, agave, sweet potatoes, vegetable broth, red curry paste, and salt and pepper. Stir, bring to a boil and then simmer, uncovered, for 30–45 minutes.
4. Remove soup from heat and, using an immersion blender, puree the soup.
5. Place soup on low heat and add beans, peanut butter, coconut milk, and chopped cilantro leaves. Cook on low heat for an additional 5–10 minutes, stirring frequently.
6. Serve in bowls and garnish with cilantro leaves. Garnish with peanuts if desired.

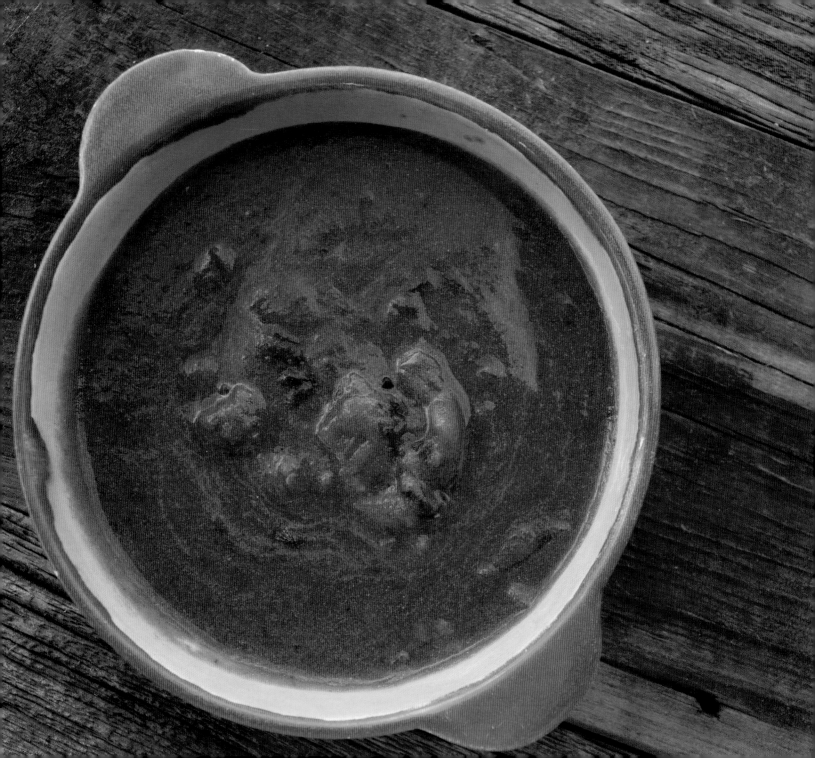

COMMUNITY CREAMY TOMATO *(v)*

If available to you, why not use tomatoes that are canned from your local community garden? Just as we may be able to tell when food is made with love, we may be able to sense, through our foods, when a community comes together to benefit friends, family, and neighbors. Our friend and Chicago-based chef, Nathan, taught us that we may freeze tomatoes from our gardens at the end of the growing season and use them year-round for soups and sauces. Just run the thawed tomatoes under water and the skin will come right off. Dice and they are ready to use. Serves 4–5.

    2T olive oil
    1 medium white onion (chopped)
    4 large garlic cloves (chopped)
    1 cup basil (chopped)
    10–12 medium (diced) or 28 oz. chopped tomatoes with juices
    ¼ cup tomato paste
    Very small pinch of saffron threads (optional)
    1½ cups vegetable broth
    2T agave nectar
    Dash of cayenne pepper
    Himalayan salt coarsely ground (to taste)
    Pepper coarsely ground (to taste)
    Cheesecloth purse (with 2 sprigs of thyme, 2 sprigs of oregano, and 2 bay leaves)
    ¼ cup heavy cream (optional)
    Basil leaves (garnish)

1. In a large saucepan or Dutch oven over medium heat, sauté onion and garlic in olive oil until softened or for about 5 minutes.
2. Add basil and sauté for an additional 2–3 minutes.
3. To saucepan, add tomatoes, tomato paste, saffron, vegetable broth, agave, cayenne, salt, pepper, and cheesecloth purse.
4. Bring ingredients to a boil and then simmer for 15–20 minutes.
5. Remove soup from heat and discard cheesecloth purse. Use an immersion blender to blend soup.
6. Add heavy cream, stirring frequently.
7. Ladle soup in bowls and garnish with basil leaves.

THE RIVER YOGA COMMUNITY

"There are only two lasting bequests we can hope to give our children. One of these is roots; the other, wings."
W. HODDING CARTER

River Yoga is a yoga and wellness center based in the Thousand Islands, New York, which is an incredibly special place that draws students from around the world. River Yoga encourages and empowers each student to discover his or her individual practice and unique path toward whole health and is embraced for its all-level, school-age, and chair programs. Ultimately, River Yoga is a place where you simply *are*. River Yoga is continually strengthened by its students' inspirational practices on and, more importantly, off of their mats.

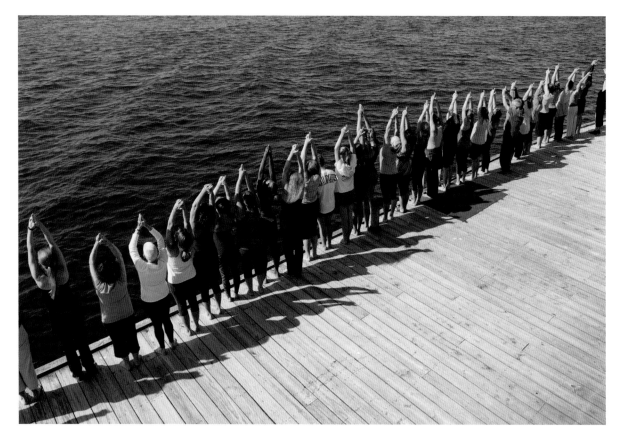

Uttarabodhi Mudra • Hand Gesture Representing Enlightenment

HARMONY

"Yoga is like music. The rhythm of the body, the melody of the mind and the harmony of the soul create the symphony of life."
B.K.S. IYENGAR

Just as we do not listen to a song to hear it reach its end, we do not come to our mat to reach the end of our practice.

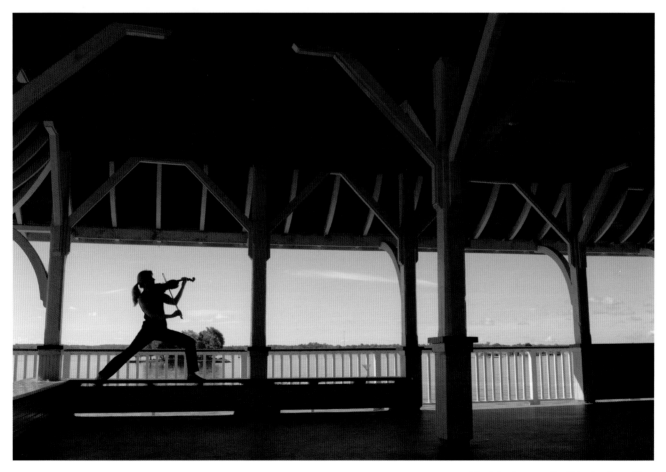

Virabhadrasana II • Warrior Pose Two

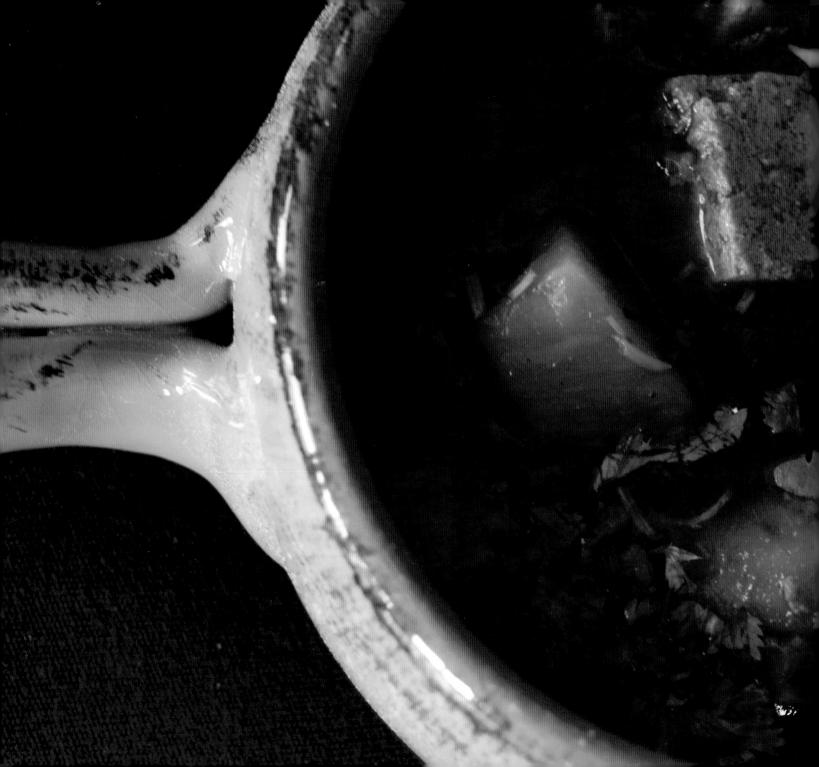

HATHA HOT & SOUR (v)

Hatha (ha = sun, tha = moon) yoga is a type of yoga that focuses on postures that explore and create balance among opposing forces. Hatha yoga helps us to focus on our breath through a moving meditation of postures. The practice ultimately helps us to strengthen the connection between mind, body, and inner spirit. Our Hatha Hot & Sour soup combines a variety of ingredients with exceptional textural and taste experiences. We hope you enjoy this healthy, well-balanced soup. Serves 8–10.

4 cups Asian dried mushrooms
6 cups water
2T olive oil
1 medium white onion (thinly sliced)
3T fresh ginger (minced)
3 scallions (greens removed and sliced)
2T lemongrass (thinly sliced)
¼ cup tamari
1T chili paste
¼ cup rice vinegar
2T agave nectar
10 oz. frozen super firm tofu (thawed, liquid squeezed out, and cut into ½-inch cubes)
1 cup fresh pineapple (cut into ½-inch cubes)
½ cup cilantro leaves (loosely chopped)
2T basil leaves (chopped into thin slices)

1. Reconstitute mushrooms in 6 cups of hot water until tender (this may take 30 minutes to 1 hour). Remove from water, drain, and reserve mushroom water. Thinly slice mushrooms. Set aside.
2. In large saucepan or Dutch oven over medium heat, sauté onion, ginger, scallions, and lemongrass in olive oil for about 5–10 minutes.
3. Add tamari, chili paste, rice vinegar, agave, sliced mushrooms, reserved mushroom water, tofu, and pineapple. Bring soup to a boil and then simmer for about 30 to 45 minutes.
4. Turn heat off and stir in cilantro and basil. Allow soup to rest for 5 minutes.
5. Serve in bowls. Enjoy!

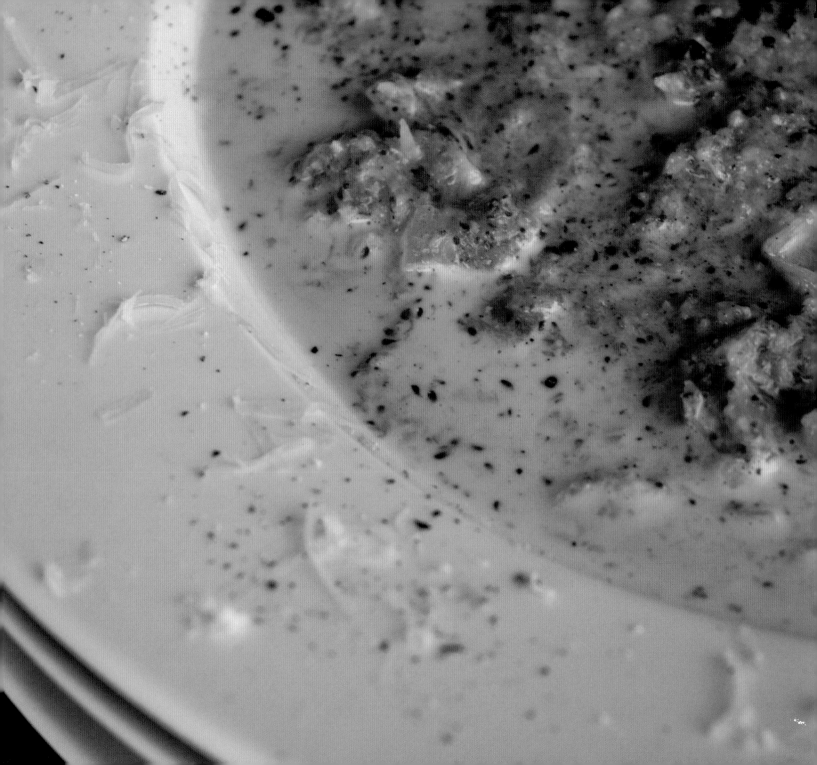

CHEDDAR CHI & BROCCOLI

While in the Western world we often use the word "breath" to explain the act of inhalation and exhalation, many Eastern cultures take the word "breath" one step further, emphasizing that breath is our "life force" or "breath of life." As noted previously, the Sanskrit word "prana" means "life force." The Chinese word for "life force" is "chi." As we breathe fully through our eating and yoga practices we become more present, savoring our experiences. Broccoli is a wonderfully healthful vegetable, as it is packed with vitamins and minerals that may lower the risk of developing a number of diseases. Our Cheddar Chi & Broccoli soup is a lovely way to end the day. Serves 8–10.

2 large heads of broccoli
1T olive oil
1 medium white onion (chopped)
½ cup canned green chilies
2 medium garlic cloves (chopped)
¼ tsp. ground nutmeg
¼ tsp. ground cinnamon
½ tsp. ground cumin
Dash of cayenne pepper
½ tsp. ground turmeric
Himalayan salt coarsely ground (to taste)
Black pepper ground (to taste)
4 cups vegetable broth
2 cups extra sharp cheddar cheese, shredded *(we use River Rat XXX Sharp)*

1. Cut stalks off of broccoli and roughly chop florets.
2. In a large saucepan or Dutch oven, sauté onion, chilies, and garlic in olive oil for 5 minutes over medium heat. Add broccoli florets, spices, salt, pepper, broth, and cheese. Bring to a boil and then simmer for about 30 minutes, stirring occasionally. Use an immersion blender if desired to make soup smoother in consistency.
3. Ladle into bowls and serve. Enjoy!

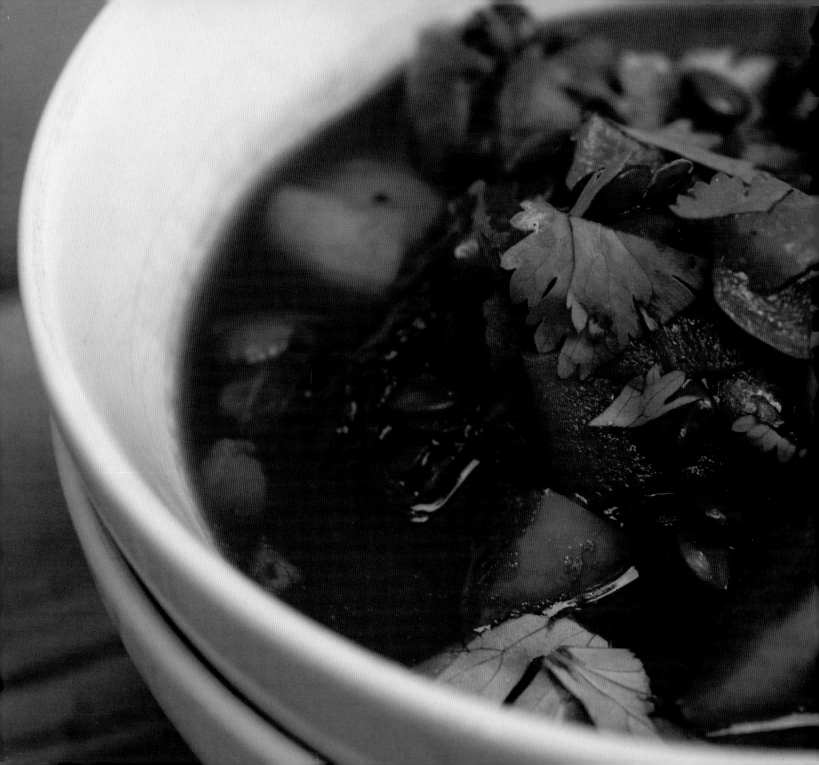

LIBERATING LENTIL (v)

Set your other lentil soup recipes free and allow yourself to revel in this unique and totally divine lentil soup. Our Liberating Lentil soup contains mustard greens, apple, lentils (of course), and a bevy of nutritional spices. Mustard greens contain Vitamin K, which promotes bone health. Lentils are nutty and earthy in flavor and support digestive and heart health. This is a hearty vegan soup. Serves 4.

2T olive oil
2 medium garlic cloves (chopped)
2T fresh ginger (minced)
1 medium white onion (chopped)
2 cups mustard greens (or other dark greens de-ribbed and torn into 1-inch pieces)
1 cup tart apple (chopped)
1 tsp. ground mustard
½ tsp. ground turmeric
½ tsp. ground cumin
Dash of cayenne pepper
¼ tsp. ground nutmeg
¼ tsp. ground cinnamon
Himalayan salt coarsely ground (to taste)
Pepper coarsely ground (to taste)
1T brown sugar
5 cups vegetable broth
2T tomato paste
2 cups lentils
½ cup fresh cilantro (chopped)

1. In a large saucepan or Dutch oven, sauté garlic, ginger, and white onion in olive oil for about 5 minutes over medium heat.
2. Add greens, apple, ground mustard, turmeric, cumin, cayenne, nutmeg, cinnamon, salt, and pepper. Stir to combine and cook for an additional 3 minutes.
3. Stir in brown sugar, vegetable broth, tomato paste, and lentils. Bring to a boil and then simmer for 30 minutes to 1 hour (or until lentils are al dente).
4. Turn the heat off and add the cilantro. Let the soup sit for about 10 minutes. Ladle the soup into bowls and serve.

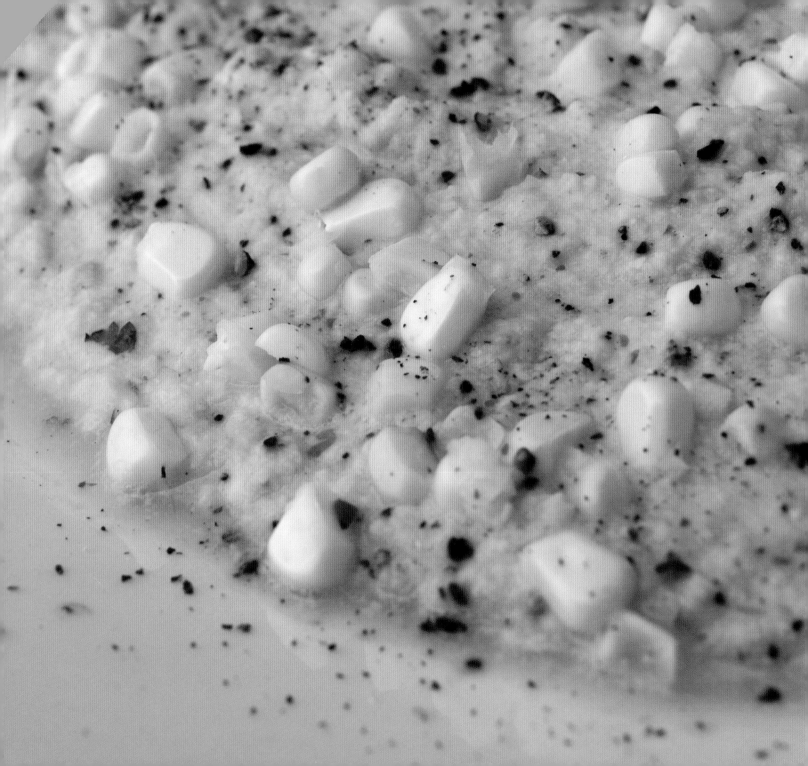

RAW DEAL: CASHEW CORN CHOWDER *(v)(r)*

This is a fun, easy raw soup to try as an avid or new connoisseur of raw food. Raw food is typically not cooked over 115°F and it is unprocessed. People who follow raw diets do so, in part, because a significant amount of foods' nutritional values are lost when heated above 115°F. We know many people, including dairy and meat eaters, who think this is, hands down, the best corn chowder they've ever had. We agree! Serves 4–6.

5 cups fresh yellow corn
1 cup water
2 cups raw cashews
4T olive oil
2 medium garlic cloves
¼ tsp. cumin
½ jalapeño (seeded and de-ribbed)
2 small tomatoes
Himalayan salt coarsely ground (to taste)
Pepper coarsely ground (to taste)
2T fresh cilantro leaves (chopped, plus leaves for garnish)

1. In a blender combine 3½ cups of corn with water, cashews, olive oil, garlic, cumin, jalapeño, tomatoes, salt, pepper, and chopped cilantro leaves.
2. Pour into a large soup bowl and stir in remaining 1½ cups of corn.
3. Place in individual serving bowls and garnish with cilantro leaves. Serve at room temperature.

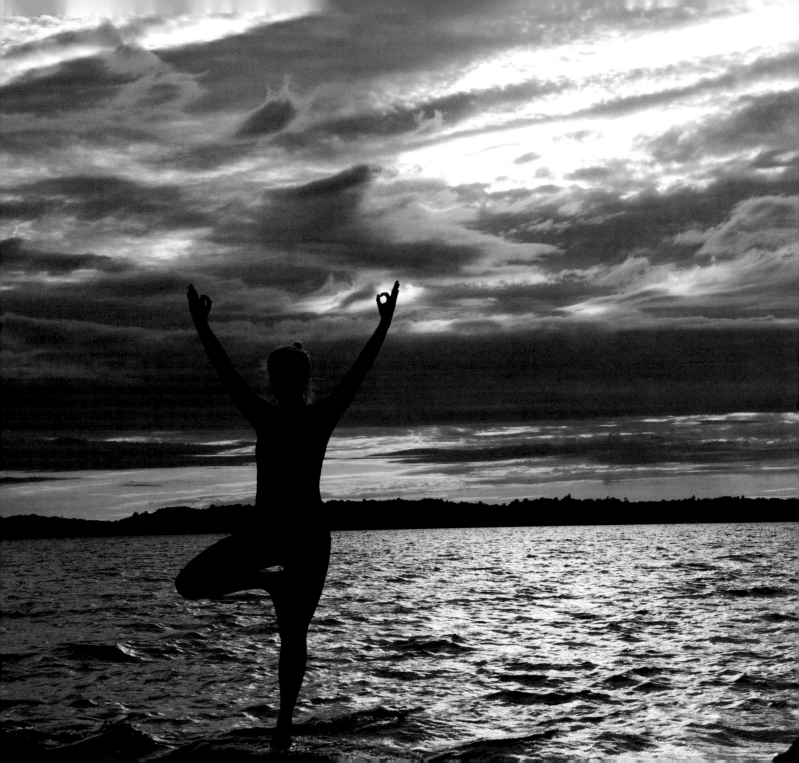

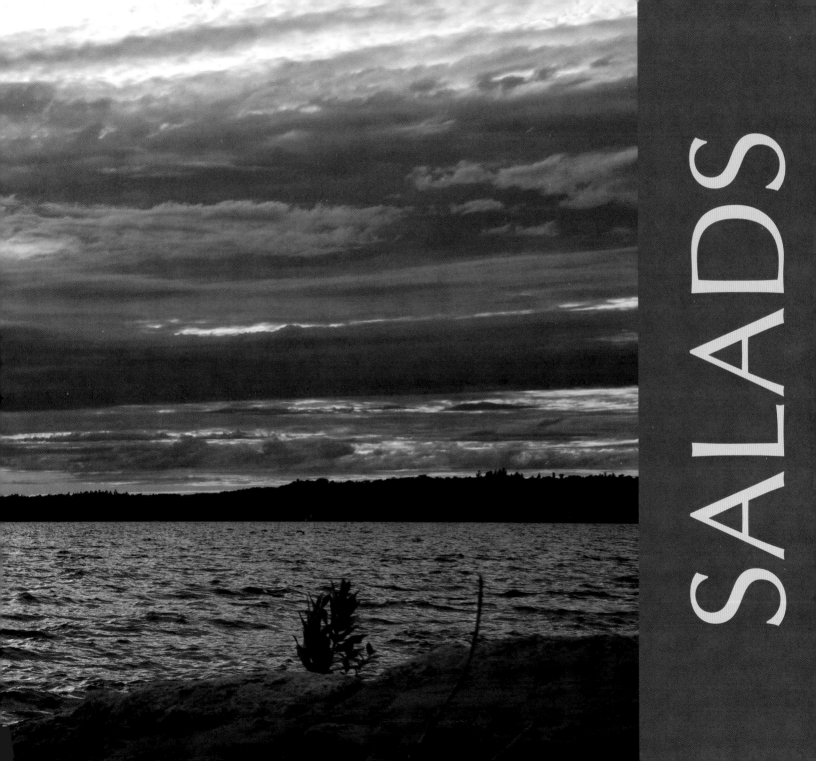

SALADS

INTENTION INGREDIENTS

When we set an intention—explore, gratitude, nourish, surrender, taste, authenticity, bliss, patience, savor, awaken—we send a message out to the universe. When we focus our attention on our intention, we realize what we want or need.

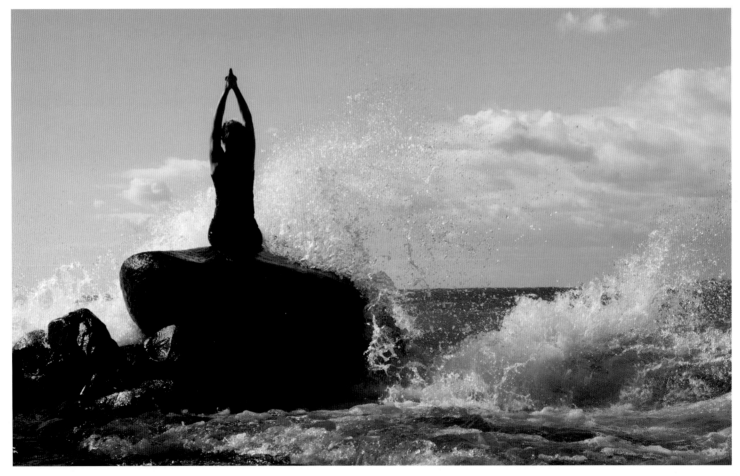

Uttarabodhi Mudra • Hand Gesture Representing Enlightenment

INTENTION / ATTENTION

"When you live your life with an appreciation of coincidences and their meanings, you connect with the underlying field of infinite possibilities."
DEEPAK CHOPRA

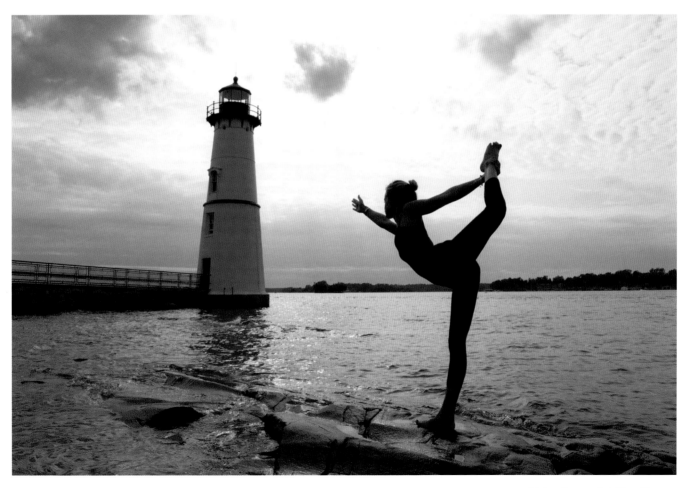

Natarajasana II • King Dancer

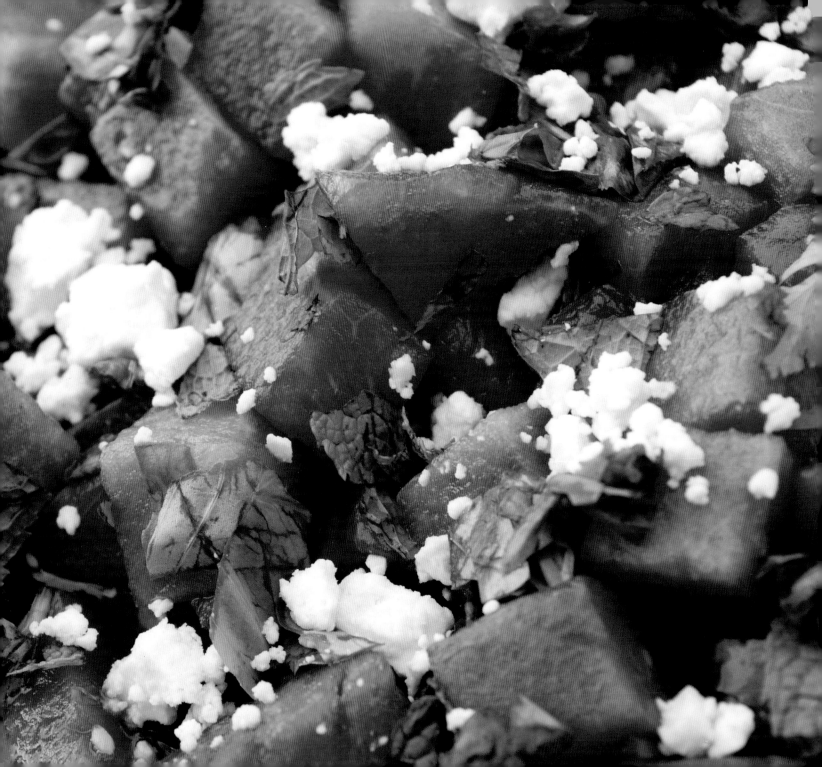

INTENTION-INFUSED WATERMELON *(v)*

Before making this recipe, set an intention for the preparation or enjoyment of the meal. Your intention may be as simple as "joy." Embrace your intention and be aware of how you feel as well as how that may affect those around you. Our intention for creating this Intention-Infused Watermelon salad was "relish"; we aimed to create a healthy dish that all of our family members would appreciate and enjoy. We hope you do as well! Serves 10 as an appetizer.

½ cup water
¼ cup brown sugar
½ cup balsamic vinegar
½ watermelon cut into 1-inch-thick cubes
¼ cup feta cheese (optional)
¼ cup fresh basil (chopped into thin slices)
2T fresh mint (chopped into thin slices)

1. Place water, brown sugar, and balsamic vinegar in a small saucepan over medium heat. Stir until sugar dissolves. Remove from heat and let mixture rest until it reaches room temperature.
2. Place cubed watermelon into a large bowl. Cover with vinegar mixture and chill in refrigerator for at least 4 hours, stirring once an hour.
3. Remove from refrigerator and place about 8 cubes on each plate. Top each cube with a pinch of feta cheese, basil, and mint slices.

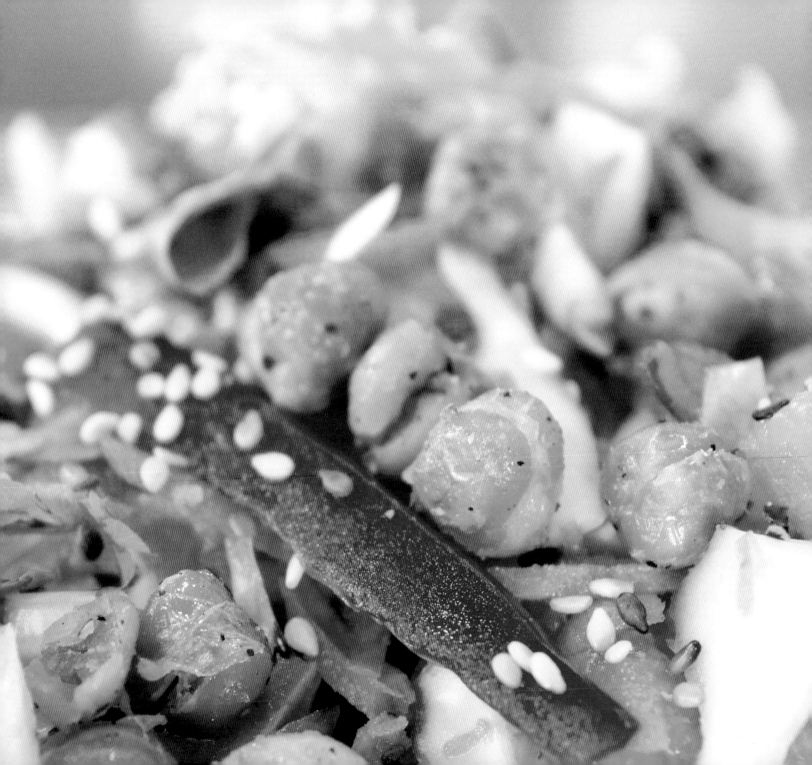

COURAGEOUSLY CHOPPED (v)

The origin of the English word "courage" comes from the French word "coeur," which means heart. Our yoga practices will guide us to the realization that the answers we seek come from within. With courage and an open heart we are guided to act truthfully and kindly. Our Courageously Chopped salad is our variation of an Asian chopped salad. It will leave you satiated and ready to take on new adventures (with an open heart)! Serves 8–10 as an appetizer.

Not-So-Plain Chicks (see recipe on page 20)

1 cup *Yummy Yin dressing* (see recipe on page 158)

4T sesame seeds

2 cups romaine lettuce (thinly chopped)
2 cups green or red cabbage (shredded)
1 cup carrot (shredded)
1 red pepper (seeded, de-ribbed, and thinly sliced)
1 cup mandarin oranges (drained)
½ cup scallion (chopped)
½ cup cilantro (chopped)

1. Prepare *Not-So-Plain Chicks* and *Yummy Yin* dressing recipes.
2. In a medium skillet over low-medium heat, toast sesame seeds until golden brown and fragrant. Remove from heat and set aside.
3. Combine romaine, cabbage, carrot, red pepper, oranges, scallion, and cilantro.
4. Combine salad with *Yummy Yin* dressing.
5. Top with *Not-So-Plain Chicks* and toasted sesame seeds.
6. Serve immediately.

COURAGE

"Your time is limited, so don't waste it living someone else's life. Don't be trapped by dogma—which is living with the results of other people's thinking. Don't let the noise of others' opinions drown out your own inner voice. And most important, have the courage to follow your heart and intuition."
STEVE JOBS

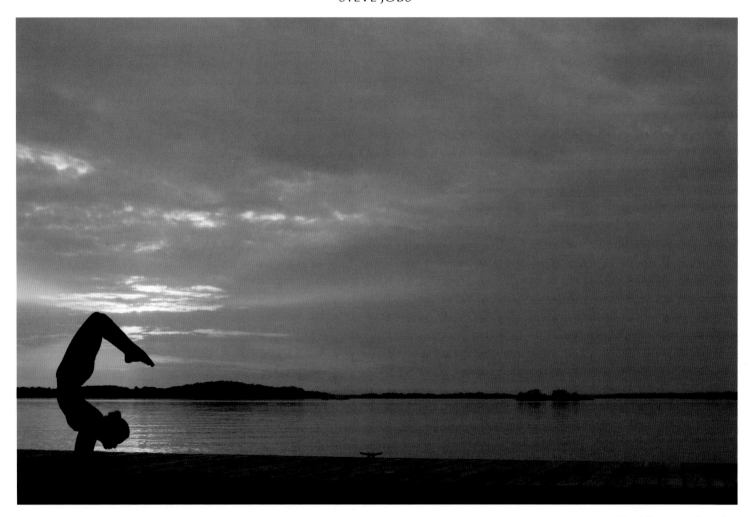

Vrschikasana • Scorpion

KARMA

"People ask me what my religion is. I tell them, my religion is kindness."
HIS HOLINESS THE XIV DALAI LAMA

Karma is the law of cause and effect. Embrace the opportunity to say what makes you feel joyful.
Your joyfulness will impact the joyfulness of others, and will again
find its way back to you.

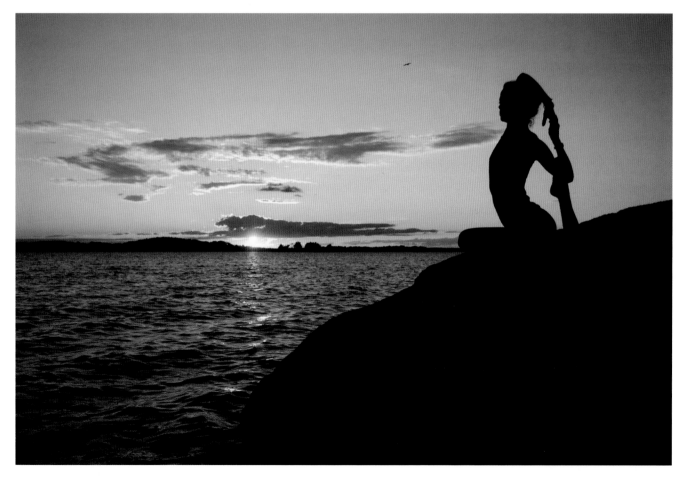

Eka Pada Rajakapotasana III • Royal Pigeon Posture

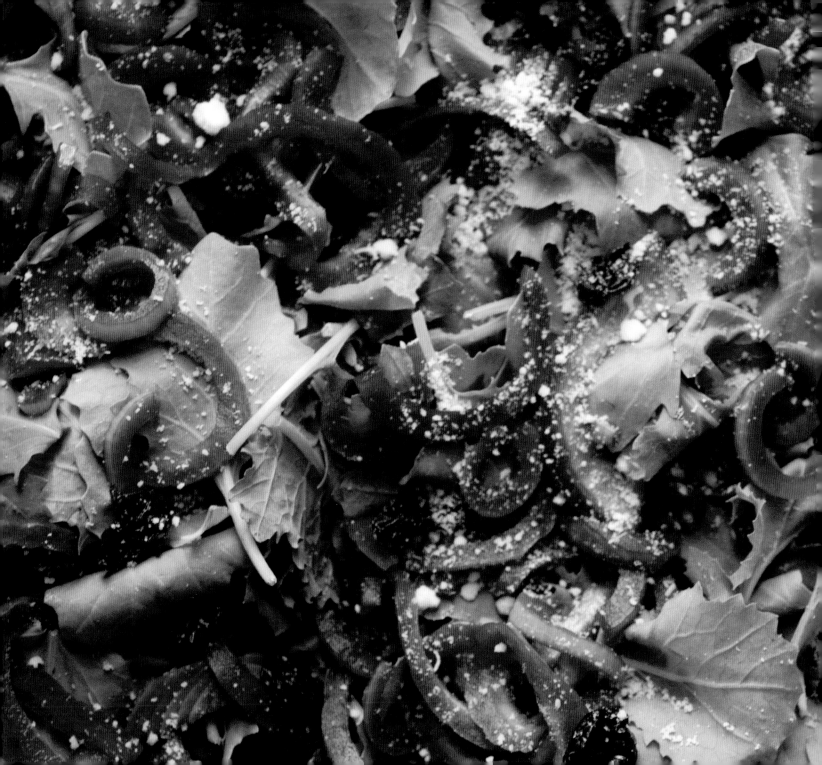

KARMA KALE CAESAR *(v)*

Karma originates from the Sanskrit word "karman," which basically translates to "action, effect, fate." This means what you do or what you have done will produce an effect for your future. So, our thinking is by making mindful, healthy choices, including the foods we eat, we embrace a healthy future. One healthy choice—eating kale! Kale is rich in vitamin A, vitamin C, and other antioxidants. Baby kale will have a less prickly texture and is nice to use when available. The dressing for this salad is our Cobra Caesar, called such because of its strong garlic and lemon notes. It is delightfully bold and pairs nicely with the kale. Serves 6–8 as an appetizer.

1 cup red wine vinegar
⅓ cup water
½ cup brown sugar (packed)
Himalayan salt coarsely ground (to taste)
1 cup red onion (thinly sliced)
6–8 cups raw kale
½ cup dried cherries

1 cup *Cobra Caesar* dressing (see recipe on page 160)

1. Combine vinegar, water, brown sugar, and salt in a medium saucepan. Bring to a boil over medium-high heat until sugar dissolves. Immediately pour vinegar mixture over onions and combine. Let mixture rest and cool for at least 20 minutes.
2. Use a salad spinner to clean and dry kale thoroughly. De-rib kale by tearing leaves off of large stalks into 1-inch pieces.
3. Prepare *Cobra Caesar* dressing.
4. Pour liquid off of onions. Combine pickled onions, cherries, and kale. Combine ingredients with dressing.
5. Serve immediately.

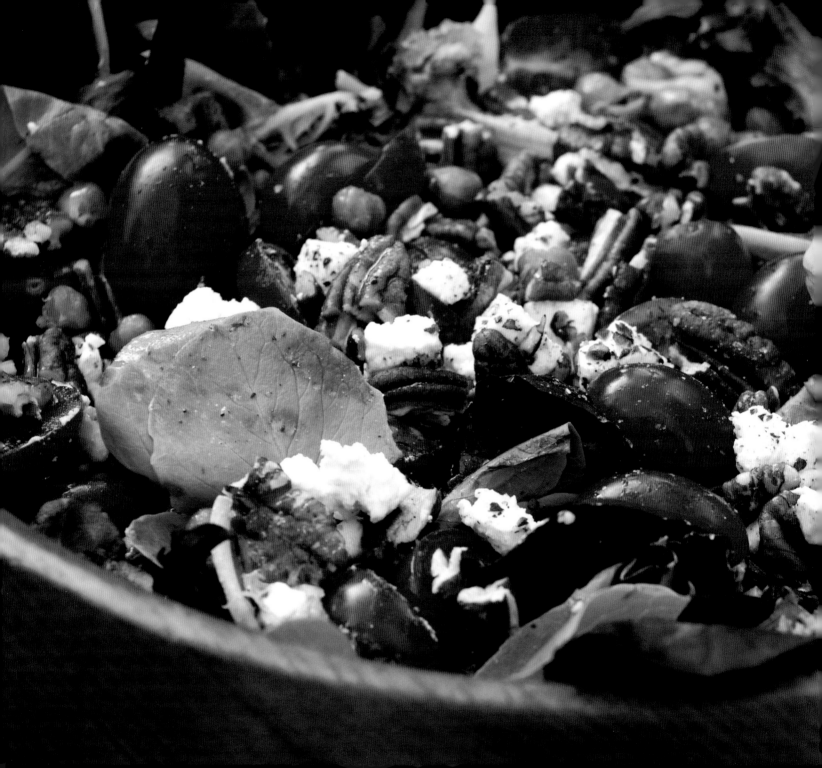

YUM, YUM, YUM *(v)*

The Sanskrit word "yam"—which is often pronounced "yum"—is a mantra used to help open the heart chakra. Deepak Chopra and Oprah Winfrey offer a guided meditation, encouraging people to repeat the words—"Yum, Yum, Yum"—to help send a ripple of peace and abundance into the world. The play-on-words title of this recipe as well as our company name (Live Yum) stemmed from this lesson. Thank you Deepak and Oprah. Your vision and your work are an inspiration to us. Our Yum, Yum, Yum salad was the first recipe we included in this book and is very special to us for the reasons outlined above (plus, it's completely yummy). Thank you for inviting us into your kitchens and sharing this experience. Serves 6–8 as an appetizer.

½ cup raw pecans
Himalayan salt coarsely ground (to taste)

Not-So-Plain Chicks (see recipe on page 20)

Yum, Yum, Yum dressing (see recipe on page 144)

4 cups mixed greens
½ cup goat cheese, crumbled (optional)
½ cup cherry tomatoes (cut in half lengthwise)

1. Toast pecans in a medium skillet over low-medium heat, adding salt to taste throughout process, until golden brown and fragrant. Remove from heat and set aside.
2. Prepare *Not-So-Plain Chicks* and *Yum, Yum, Yum* dressing.
3. Combine greens, goat cheese, tomatoes, and *Yum, Yum, Yum* dressing in a large salad bowl. Top with *Not-So-Plain Chicks* and toasted pecans.
4. Serve immediately.

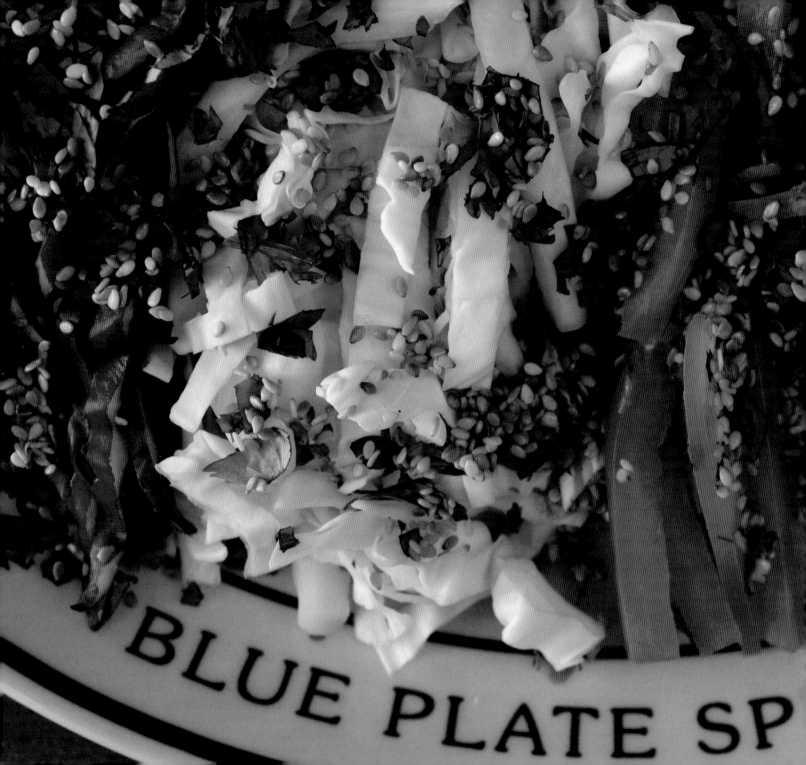

CHAKRA VEGETABLE SLAW *(v)(r)*

Chakras are energy centers in the body through which energy flows. Our bodies host seven major chakras and each chakra is associated with a different color—Root (Red), Sacral (Orange), Solar Plexus (Yellow), Heart (Green), Throat (Blue), Third Eye (Indigo), and Crown (Violet). Our Chakra Vegetable Slaw (with the presentation on a blue plate) represents the seven chakra colors found in our bodies. It's a fun way to present a slaw and ignite a chakra conversation among your dining companions. For a raw version, do not toast the sesame seeds. Serves 8–10 as an appetizer.

1 cup *Ginger Glow* dressing (see recipe on page 158)

½ cup sesame seeds
1 cup red pepper (shredded)
1 cup carrot (shredded)
1 cup yellow pepper (shredded)
1 cup green cabbage (shredded)
1 blue plate (for serving)
1 cup radicchio or red cabbage (shredded)
½ cup cilantro (chopped)

1. Prepare *Ginger Glow* dressing. Set aside.
2. Toast sesame seeds in a medium skillet over low-medium heat until golden brown and fragrant. Set aside.
3. Arrange shredded vegetables on a blue plate in the order of the chakras (above) starting with the red pepper at the bottom of the plate and ending with the radicchio at the top of the plate. Sprinkle with toasted sesame seeds and cilantro.
4. Before serving, combine slaw with dressing.

FREEDOM

Lokah Samastah Sukhino Bhavantu
"May all beings everywhere be happy and free, and may the thoughts, words, and actions of my own life contribute in some way to that happiness and to that freedom for all."

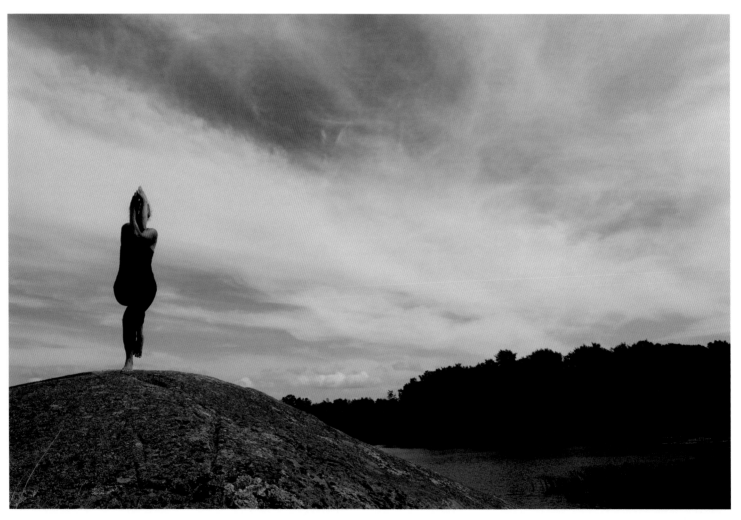

Garudasana • Eagle Pose

ENERGY

Our yoga practices have the abilities to empower us mentally, embolden us emotionally, strengthen us physically, and purify us consciously.

Why would we want anything different from our food?

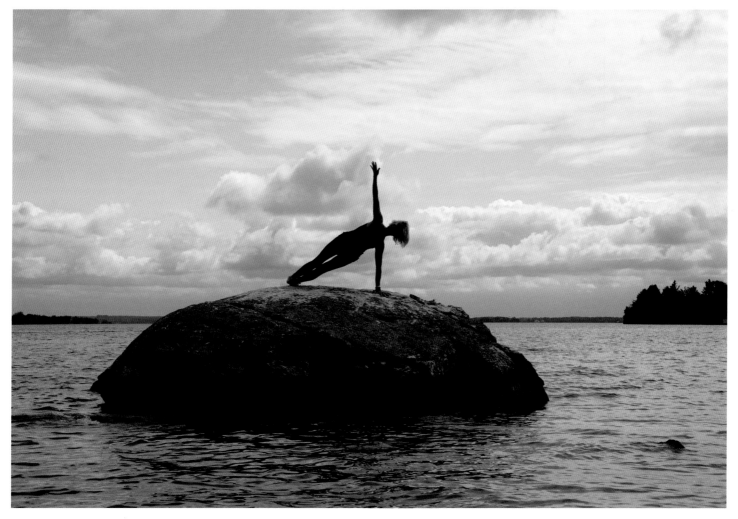

Vasisthasana II • Side Plank

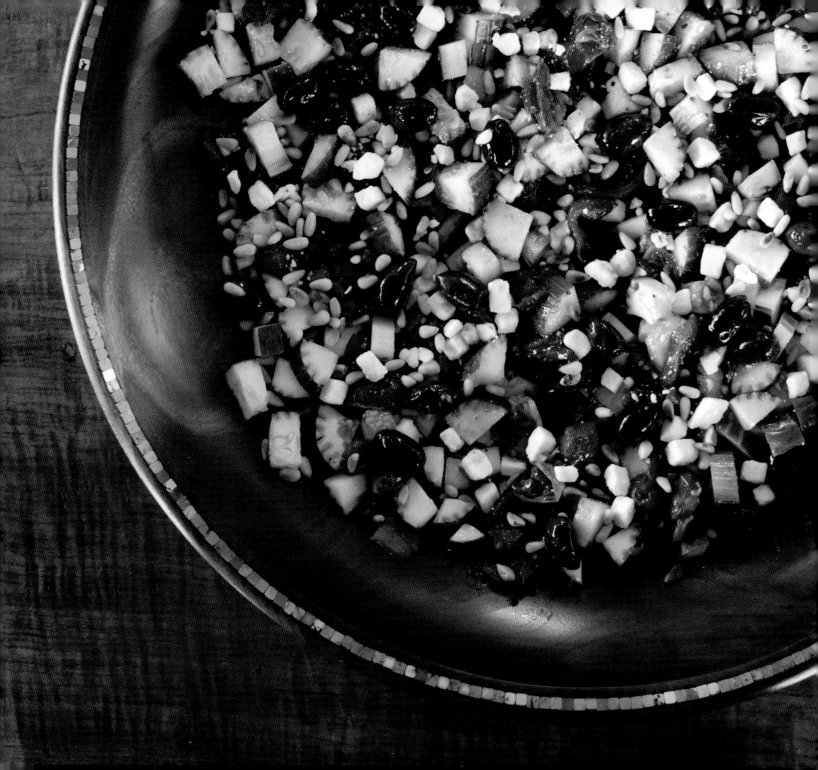

HUMBLE HERO *(v)*

Our version of a classic Greek salad is served family style and uses our Realized Roasted Tomatoes. The "family style" of serving is a great way to share a dining experience with family or friends. The dish serves as a conversation piece from its presentation, during the meal, and even while cleaning up. In our conversations, we like to be mindful that it is important to listen to the student and teacher within all of us. Serves 8–10 as an appetizer.

Realized Roasted Tomatoes (see recipe on page 68)

½ cup pine nuts
½ cup basil (chopped, plus large leaves for garnish)
½ cup olive oil
¼ cup balsamic vinegar
1T agave nectar
Himalayan salt coarsely ground (to taste)
Pepper coarsely ground (to taste)
2 cups cucumber (chopped)
½ cup crumbled feta cheese (optional)
½ cup Kalamata olives (pitted)

1. Prepare *Realized Roasted Tomatoes*. Allow to rest and slice into ½-inch strips.
2. Toast nuts in a medium skillet over low-medium heat until golden brown and fragrant. Remove from heat and set aside.
3. Combine chopped basil, olive oil, balsamic vinegar, agave, salt, and pepper to form dressing. Set aside.
4. Begin plating. Start with half of your chopped cucumber. Next layer the *Realized Roasted Tomatoes* on top of the cucumbers. Combine the remaining chopped cucumber and feta cheese and sprinkle on top of *Tomatoes*. Top with roasted pine nuts. Drizzle dressing evenly over entire dish. Garnish with Kalamata olives and basil leaves.
5. Present and serve.

VIRASANA
HERO POSE

*aids in digestion, soothes abdominal discomfort, increases flexibility
in the knees and ankles*

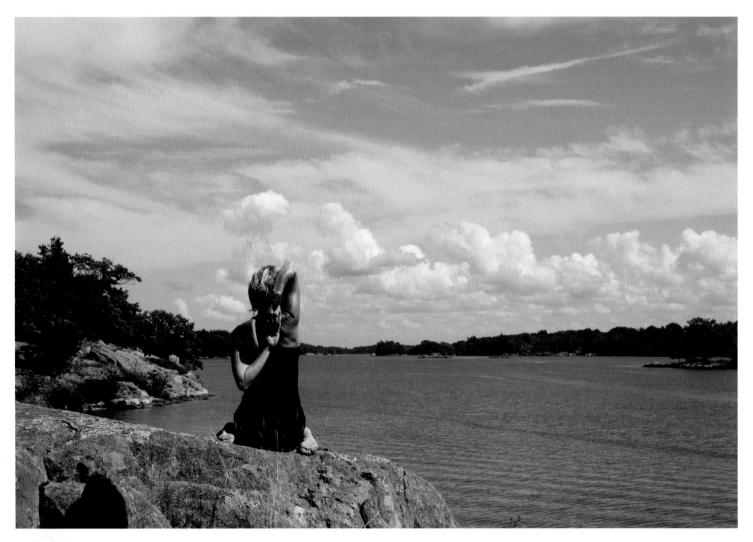

ARDHA MATSYENDRASANA
HALF LORD OF THE FISHES POSE

invigorates nervous system and massages internal organs

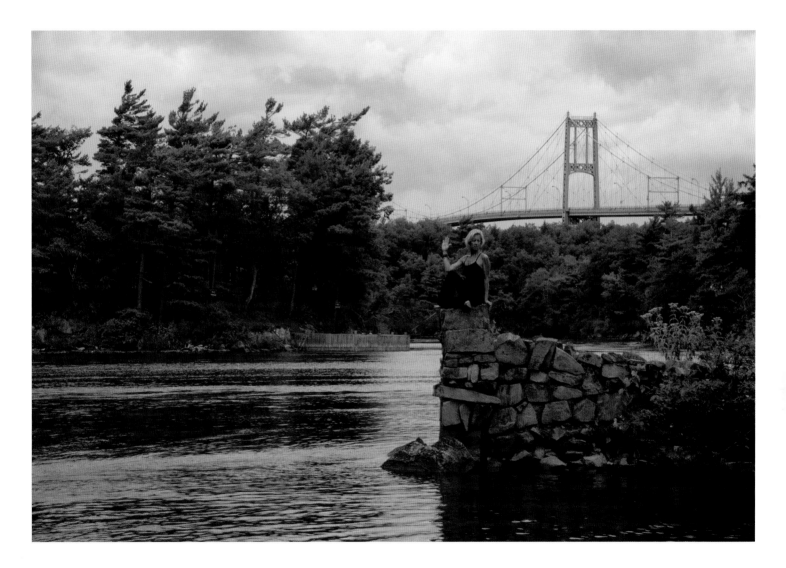

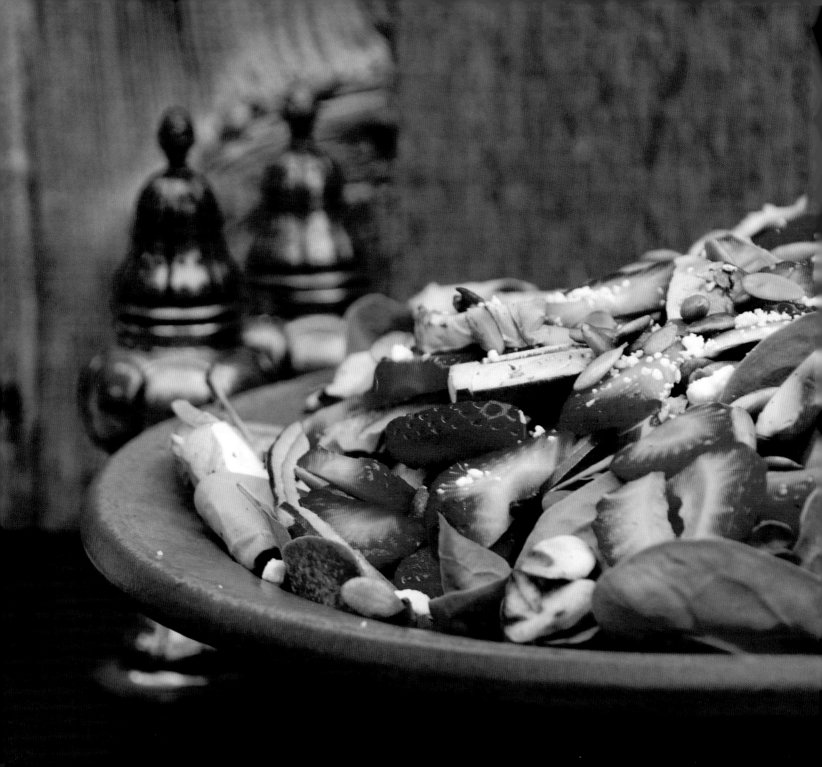

SEATED SPINACH *(v)*

Spinach packs protein, iron, vitamins, and minerals, is important for bone health, and helps to keep our skin and hair healthy. This Seated Spinach salad is dressed with our Mindful Miso dressing. Take a seat and enjoy this tasty, nutritious salad. Serves 8–10 as an appetizer.

½ cup pepitas

½ cup *Mindful Miso* dressing (see recipe on page 144)

4 cups baby spinach
4 oz. Portobello mushrooms (lightly chopped)
1 cup strawberries (thinly sliced)
¼ cup red onion (thinly sliced)
¼ cup crumbled goat cheese (optional)

1. Toast pepitas in a medium skillet over low-medium heat until golden brown and fragrant. Remove from heat and set aside.
2. Prepare *Mindful Miso* dressing.
3. Combine salad ingredients with dressing.
4. Serve immediately. Enjoy!

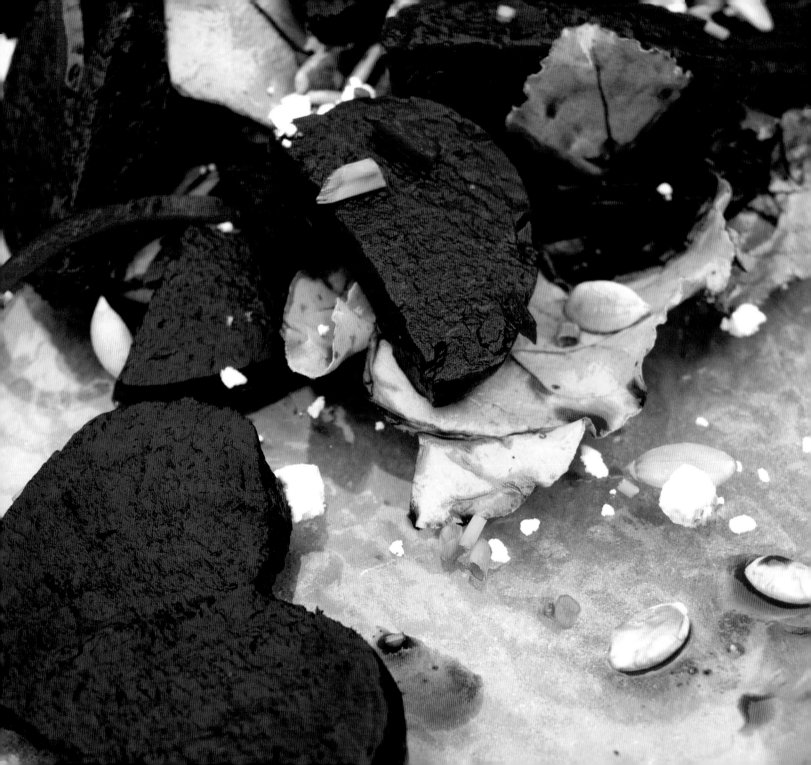

HEART"BEET" (v)

"The best and most beautiful things in the world cannot be seen or even touched—they must be felt with the heart."
HELEN KELLER

This dish was developed with love. We like to cut beet slices into the shape of hearts and place them on the top or to the side of individual serving plates as a garnish when serving. We feel this is a perfect dish to serve with a dedication to somebody you love or maybe even to somebody you don't think you love. Serves 8–10 as an appetizer.

> 2 bunches (or about 8 large) beets with beet greens intact
> 1 ½–2 cups beet greens (reserved from beet bunches)
> 1 large red onion (sliced)
> Pepper coarsely ground (to taste)
> 1 cup red wine vinegar
> ⅓ cup water
> ½ cup brown sugar (packed)
> Himalayan salt coarsely ground (to taste)
> ½ cup crumbled feta (garnish)
> ¼ cup chopped chives (garnish)
> ¼ cup pepitas (garnish)

1. Cut beet greens off of beets, leaving a 1-inch stem on beets.
2. Place beets in a large saucepan and cover by 2 inches with water. Bring water to a boil and then simmer beets in water for about 40 minutes or until fork tender. Drain the water and allow beets to cool.
3. De-rib rinsed beet greens by tearing leaves off of any large stalks and then tear greens into 2-inch pieces. Combine beet greens, red onion, and pepper in a large mixing bowl.
4. Once beets are cool, run them under water while gently removing the beet skin and stems. Slice beets into ¼- or ⅛-inch slices (save some to cut into heart shapes and serve as a garnish if desired) and place in bowl with greens and onion.
5. Combine vinegar, water, brown sugar, and salt in a medium saucepan. Bring to a boil over medium-high heat until sugar dissolves. Immediately pour vinegar mixture over beets and combine.
6. Place beets in the refrigerator overnight.
7. Toast pepitas in a skillet over low-medium heat until fragrant and golden brown. Remove from heat and set aside.
8. Before serving, top beets with feta, chives, and toasted pepitas. Garnish with heart"beets" last. Serve.

LOVE

"And in the end, the love you take is equal to the love you make."
THE BEATLES

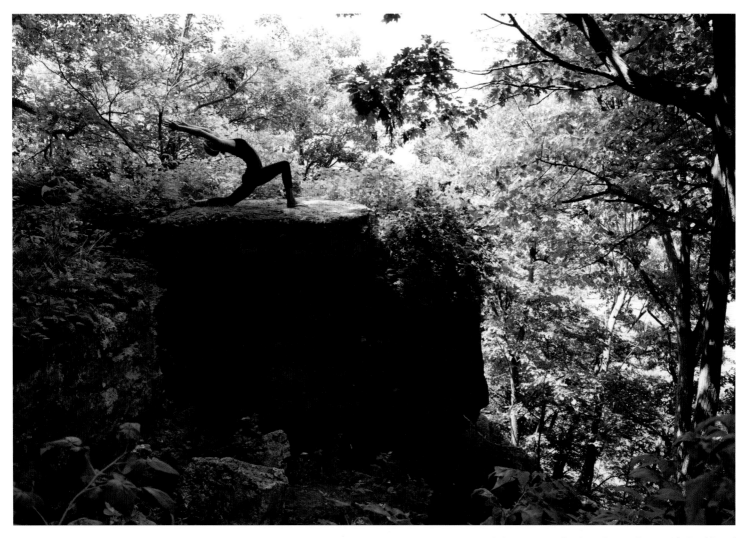

Anjaneyasana II • Low Lunge Pose with Backbend

ANANDA BALASANA
HAPPY BABY POSE

grounding, stress relieving, happiness- and laughter-inducing

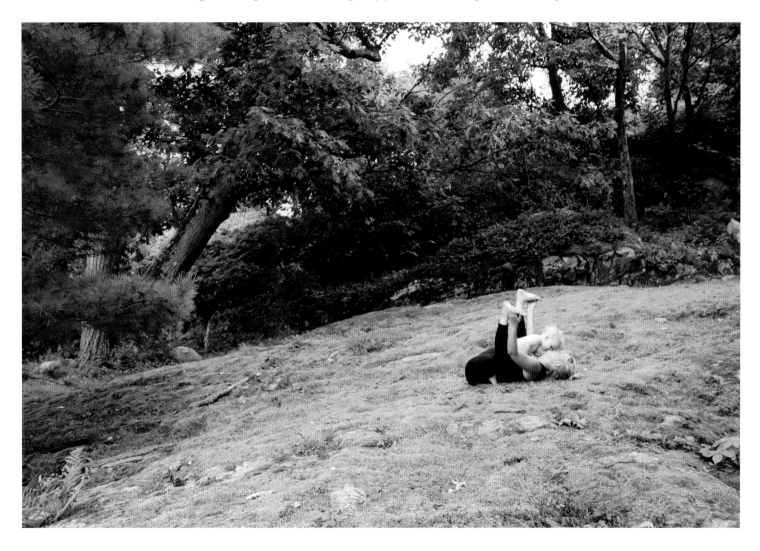

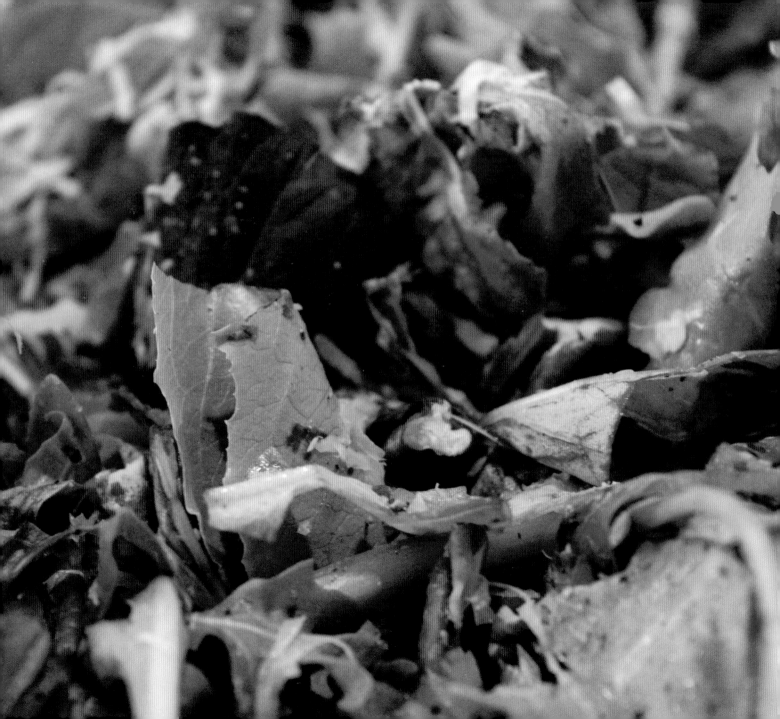

HAPPY HERB *(v)(r)*

In yoga, happiness often radiates when we are totally present in our practices, which may mean delighting in the seemingly small nuances of our postures. Our Happy Herb salad combines a variety of delicious and nutritious raw herbs and greens. The dressing for this salad is our Simplicity dressing. The key to marrying the dressing with the greens is in the preparation. Ask a partner, friend, or family member to slowly pour the Simplicity dressing over the greens while you continuously toss them with your hands. The toasted pecans balance out the lemon dressing and the Parmesan shavings add decadence to this happy, healthy, and satiating salad. Serves 8–10 as an appetizer.

½ cup raw pecans (toasting optional)
Himalayan salt coarsely ground (optional)
3 cups chopped mixed greens (spring greens, arugula, and beet greens work well)
1 cup basil (chopped)
½ cup cilantro (chopped)
¼ cup mint (chopped)
¼ cup parsley (chopped)
¼ cup dill (chopped)
½ tsp. edible lavender buds
½ cup scallion (chopped)
½ cup fresh Parmesan, shaved (optional)

Simplicity dressing (see recipe on page 154)

1. Toast pecans in a medium skillet over low-medium heat, adding salt to taste throughout process, until golden brown and fragrant. Remove from heat and set aside.
2. Combine greens, herbs, and scallions.
3. Prepare *Simplicity* dressing and dress salad.
4. Top with toasted pecans and cheese.
5. Serve immediately.

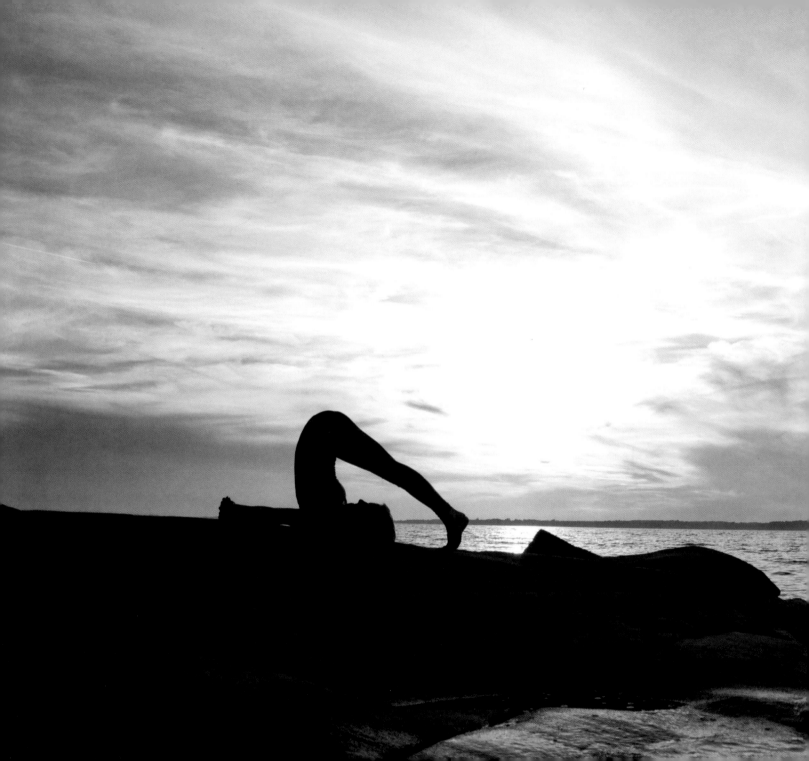

DRESSINGS & MARINADES

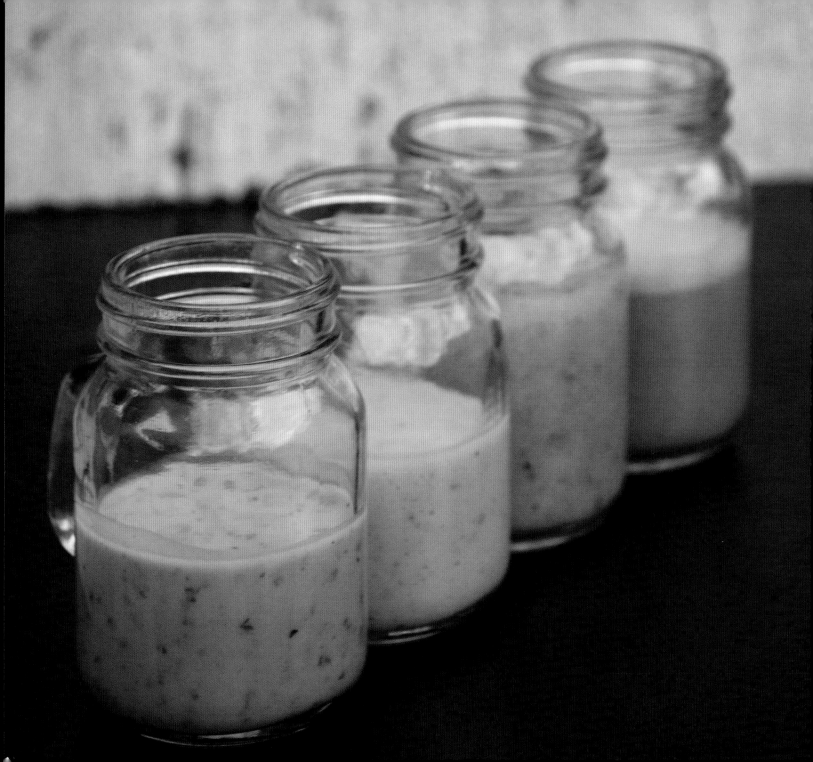

YUM, YUM, YUM (v)

Mantras—such as Yum, Yum, Yum—help us to disengage from vritti, or agitation of the mind, and ultimately, find stillness. Our Yum, Yum, Yum dressing is a versatile salad dressing that may be used on almost any favorite salad. We use this dressing with our Yum, Yum, Yum salad (see recipe on page 124). Makes about 1 cup of dressing. This dressing may be stored in the refrigerator for up to 1 week.

1T shallot (minced)
1T lime juice
3T rice vinegar
1T Dijon mustard
1T raw honey
Dash of cayenne pepper

Himalayan salt coarsely ground (to taste)
Pepper coarsely ground (to taste)
½ cup olive oil

Combine ingredients, whisking in olive oil last.

MINDFUL MISO (v)

"The present moment is filled with joy and happiness. If you are attentive, you will see it."   THICH NHAT HANH

Miso is traditionally used in Japanese cooking. It is a paste, made with fermented soybeans or other grains, that contains essential amino acids and helps to restore beneficial probiotics to the intestines. We love this dressing on our Seated Spinach salad (see recipe on page 134). Makes about 2 cups of dressing. This dressing may be stored in the refrigerator for up to 1 week.

½ cup tahini
¾ cup water
6T lemon juice
6T (white or red) miso
2T tamari
2T agave nectar
2 medium garlic cloves

Dash of ground cumin
Dash of ground cayenne pepper
Himalayan salt coarsely ground (to taste)
Pepper coarsely ground (to taste)

Combine ingredients in a food processor.

FEARLESSNESS

"Release and resolve fear, and what you want flows freely."
SHIRLEY MACLAINE

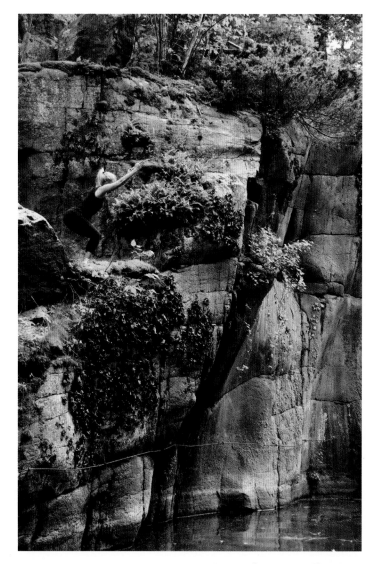

Utkatasana • Chair Pose

UTKATA KONASANA
GODDESS POSE

supports cardiovascular health, energizes the body, stimulates reproductive systems

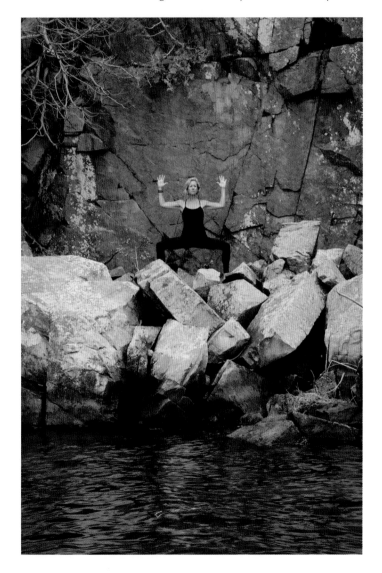

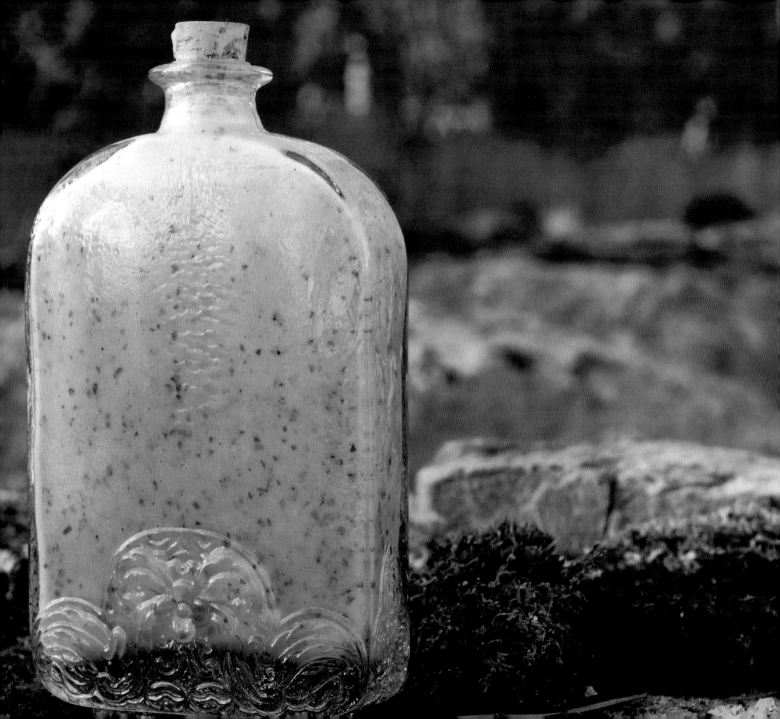

VEGAN GREEN GODDESS (v)

Three goddesses—Saraswati, Lakshmi, and Parvati—in the Hindu religion help to form the "Great Trinity." These goddesses are revered, respectively, for cosmic consciousness, wealth, and spiritual fulfillment. Ultimately, the qualities of these goddesses exist within us all. Our Vegan Green Goddess dressing is also wonderful as a marinade or dip. This recipe makes about 2 cups of dressing and may be stored in the refrigerator for up to 1 week.

4T olive oil
4T tahini
4T vegan mayonnaise
4T cider vinegar
4T tamari
2T water
4T agave
2T lemon juice
4 medium garlic cloves

2T fresh parsley
2T fresh basil
2T scallions
Himalayan salt coarsely ground (to taste)
Pepper coarsely ground (to taste)

Combine all ingredients in a food processor until smooth.

MORE THAN A THOUSAND ISLANDS (v)

One-thousand-eight-hundred-sixty-four islands to be exact. . . This dressing is a vegan variation of the traditional Thousand Islands dressing that originated where we live and love—Thousand Islands, New York. It is delicious, of course, as a dressing for salads and also works beautifully on our Reuben Revelation (see recipe on page 172). This recipe makes about 2¼ cups of dressing. It may be stored in the refrigerator for up to 1 week.

½ cup vegan mayonnaise
4T ketchup
¼ cup white wine vinegar
¼ cup orange juice
3T agave nectar
½ cup white onion (chopped)

½ cup fresh dill (chopped)
Himalayan salt coarsely ground (to taste)
Pepper coarsely ground (to taste)
Dash of cayenne pepper (to taste, optional)
½ cup olive oil
4T sweet, bread and butter–style pickles (chopped)

1. Combine mayonnaise with cayenne in food processor.
2. While ingredients are processing, slowly drizzle in olive oil.
3. Stir in chopped pickles.
4. Chill for at least 20 minutes.

SWAMI VIVEKANANDA:
FOLLOW YOUR YELLOW BRICK ROAD

*"You have to grow from the inside out. None can teach you, none can make you spiritual.
There is no other teacher but your own soul."*
SWAMI VIVEKANANDA

Swami Vivekananda—a Hindu philosopher, follower of Sri Ramakrishna, and key figure in introducing yoga to the Western world—introduced a set of meditations that he called the "Four Yogas" at the Chicago World's Fair in 1893. He described the Four Yogas as the four paths to the True Self. L. Frank Baum, author of *The Wonderful Wizard of Oz*, was listening to this speech and used the lessons from the Four Yogas to shape the goals and realizations of his characters. Scarecrow, Tin Man, Cowardly Lion, and Dorothy follow the yellow brick road searching for wisdom, compassion, courage, and inner harmony (respectively) to ultimately learn that they always possessed the qualities they were seeking.

The Thousand Islands Connection: Swami Vivekananda first traveled to the Thousand Islands, New York, in 1895 where he visited Thousand Island Park. There he cultivated his thoughts and taught his followers. To this day, monks from the Ramakrishna Order of India, known for its world-wide humanitarian efforts, and some of its millions of followers still make the pilgrimage to this very special part of the world.

FULFILLMENT

"In one word, this ideal is that you are divine."
SWAMI VIVEKANANDA

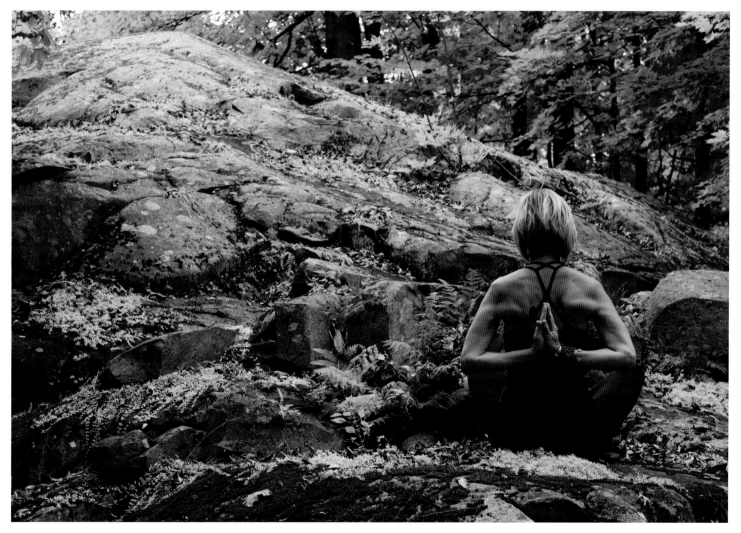

Siddhasana • Accomplished Pose with Salutation Seal

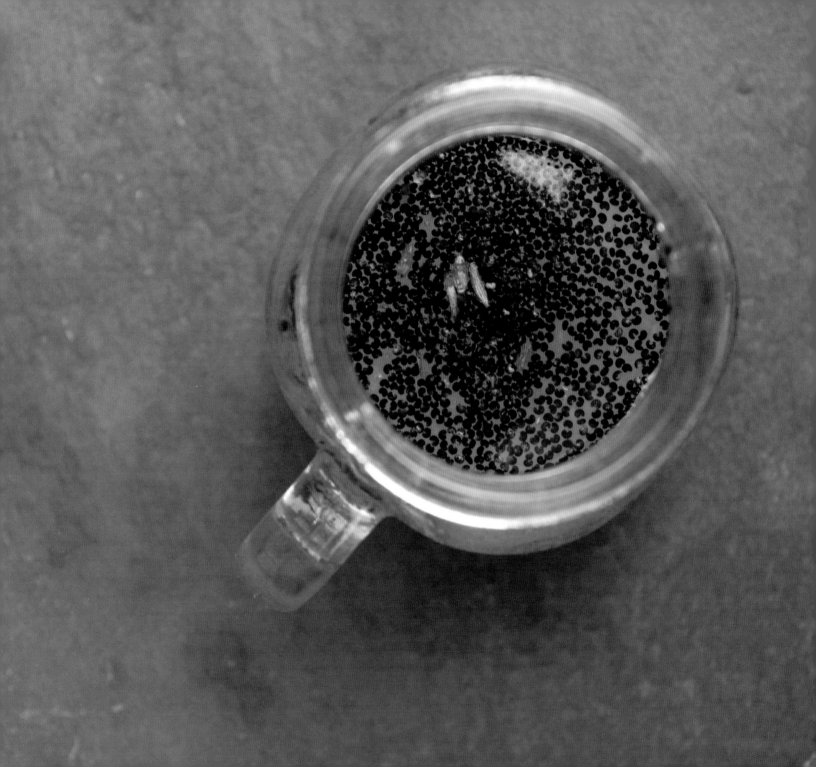

FANTASY FRUIT *(v)*

Remember that with intention and attention, fantasy may manifest into reality. . . We created this Fantasy Fruit dressing for our Chakra Fruit Salad (see recipe on page 254). It is a fun, whimsical twist for savory salads as well. Makes about ½ cup of dressing. This dressing may be stored in the refrigerator for up to 1 week.

2T raw honey
2T orange juice
2T orange zest
1T lemon juice
1 tsp. poppy seeds
1T fig paste
Small pinch of edible lavender buds (ground with fingers)

Combine ingredients.

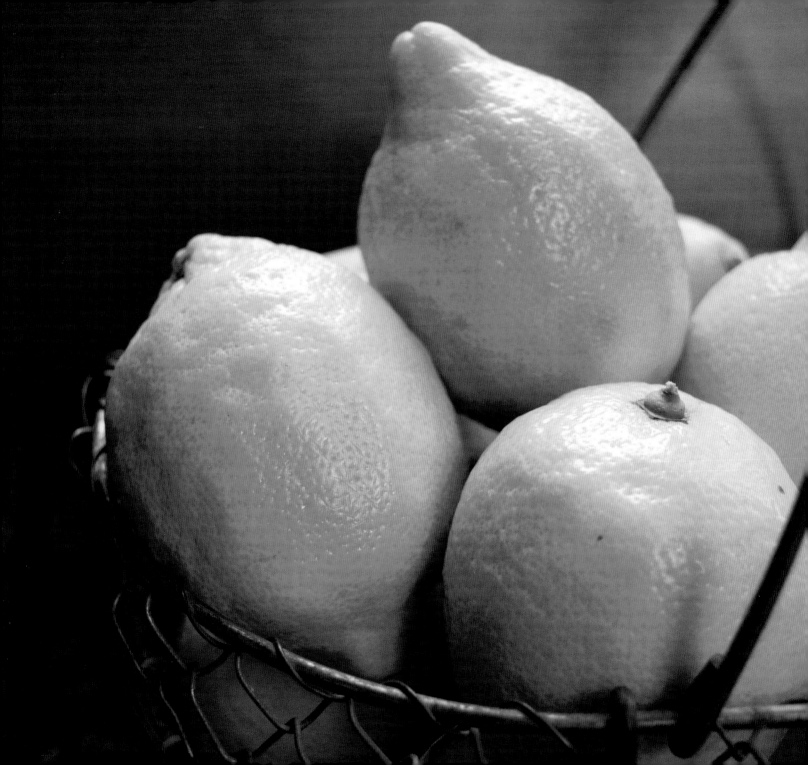

SIMPLICITY *(v)(r)*

Sometimes the most joy can be found in the simplest of things. We think that's true with this supremely easy dressing recipe. Our friend, Tim, mixes the dressing and greens with bare hands (clean, of course), which somehow makes the prepared salad even better. Thank you, Tim, for sharing this simple dressing with us! This dressing pairs beautifully with fresh herbs (try it on our Happy Herb salad, see recipe on page 140) and arugula (try it with our Awakening Arugula Svelte Pizza, see recipe on page 168).

     3T lemon juice (approximately the juice of 1 lemon)
     Himalayan salt coarsely ground (to taste)
     Pepper coarsely ground (to taste)

Combine ingredients.

SIMPLICITY

"Be content with what you have, rejoice in the way things are. When you realize there is nothing lacking, the whole world belongs to you."
LAO TZU

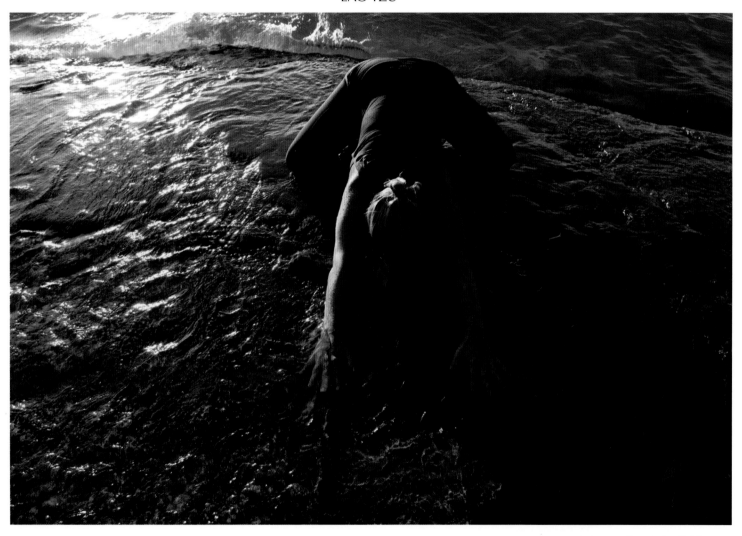

Balasana II • Wide Child's Pose

PATIENCE

"A journey of a thousand miles begins with a single step."
LAO TZU

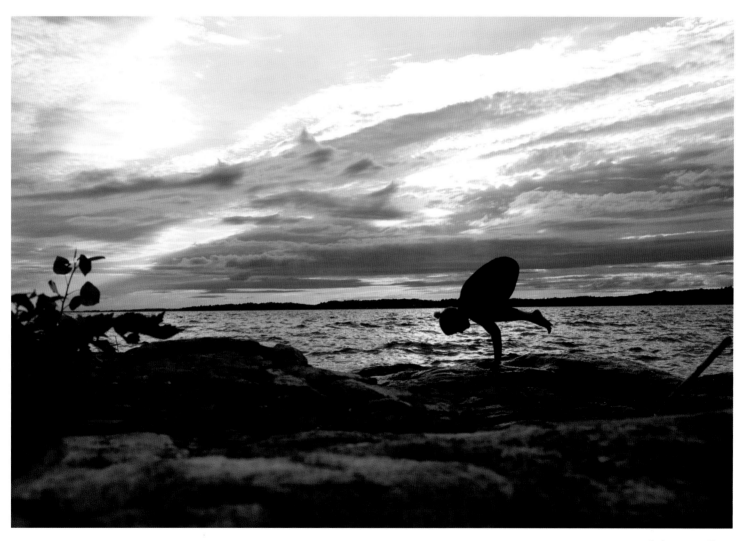

Bakasana • Crow

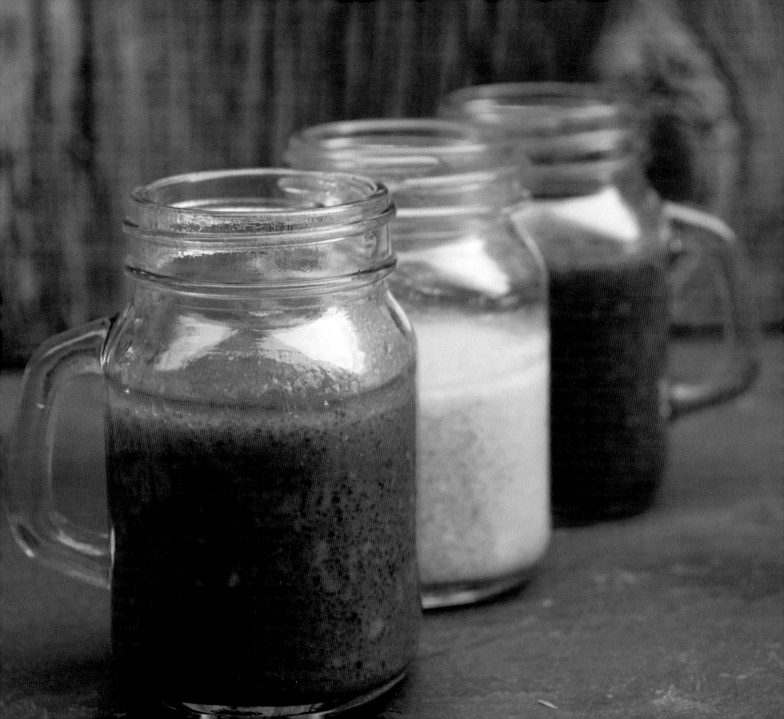

YUMMY YIN (v)

Yin Yoga is a style of yoga in which the postures are held longer to improve flexibility and also circulation in our joints. Yin Yoga poses are meant to improve the flow of energy through our chakras and thus improve our emotional, mental, and physical health. Our Yummy Yin dressing is an Asian-inspired recipe that we recommend using with our Courageously Chopped salad (see recipe on page 122).

¼ cup Hoisin sauce
¼ cup seasoned rice vinegar
2T tamari
2 medium garlic cloves (minced)
3T ginger (minced)
2T Dijon mustard
2T lime juice

1T Asian hot sauce
¼ cup olive oil
1T toasted sesame oil
Pepper coarsely ground (to taste)

Whisk ingredients together with fork until well combined.

GINGER GLOW (v)

We will admit. . . one of the benefits of yoga is getting the "yoga body." Yoga helps us to strengthen, lengthen, and tone. Yogis also often exude the "yoga glow." This glow is unique and sets yoga apart from many exercise philosophies that are not spiritually based. Yoga shines a light on our inner spirits, producing a shine from the inside out. It is this sense of inner peace and confidence that continues to shape our lifestyles and food experiences. We use this Ginger Glow recipe as a dressing and a marinade. (Sometimes we just eat it out of the mixing bowl.) It is nutritious and robust in flavor. Makes about 3 cups of dressing. This dressing may be stored in the refrigerator for up to 1 week.

1 medium yellow or Vidalia onion
2T olive oil
½ cup tamari
4T seasoned rice wine vinegar
½ cup celery

½ cup carrots
¼ cup fresh ginger
2T agave nectar
1T tomato paste
¼ tsp. Thai-style hot sauce

1. Combine ingredients in a food processor until well combined, but still slightly chunky.
2. Chill for at least 20 minutes.

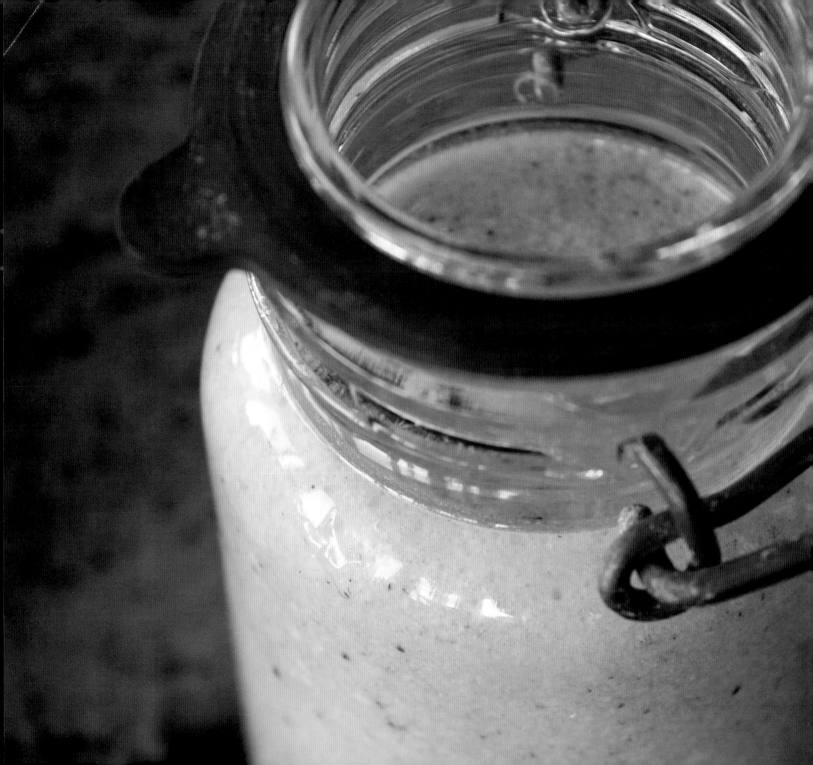

COBRA CAESAR *(v)*

Non–garlic lovers and vampires, beware! Garlic and lemon sing in this robust dressing. Though your garlic breath may not subside until the next day, garlic does boast many nutritional benefits. Used for thousands of years, garlic in your diet may reduce the risk of some cancers, fight heart disease, and serve as a potentially powerful antibiotic. We use this dressing with our Karma Kale Caesar (see recipe on page 125). Makes about 2 cups of dressing. This dressing may be stored in the refrigerator for up to 1 week.

6T lemon juice (room temperature)
4–5 medium garlic cloves (crushed)
2T Dijon mustard
1T pepper (finely ground)
½ cup olive oil
½ cup finely grated Parmesan cheese (optional)

1. Use a citrus squeezer to juice lemons. Add crushed garlic, mustard, and pepper to lemon juice. Combine.
2. Slowly whisk in olive oil.
3. Once dressing is combined, stir in Parmesan cheese.
4. Allow dressing to rest for about 30 minutes and recombine dressing if needed before mixing with greens.

BHUJANGASANA
COBRA POSE

strengthens upper body, elevates mood, opens heart center

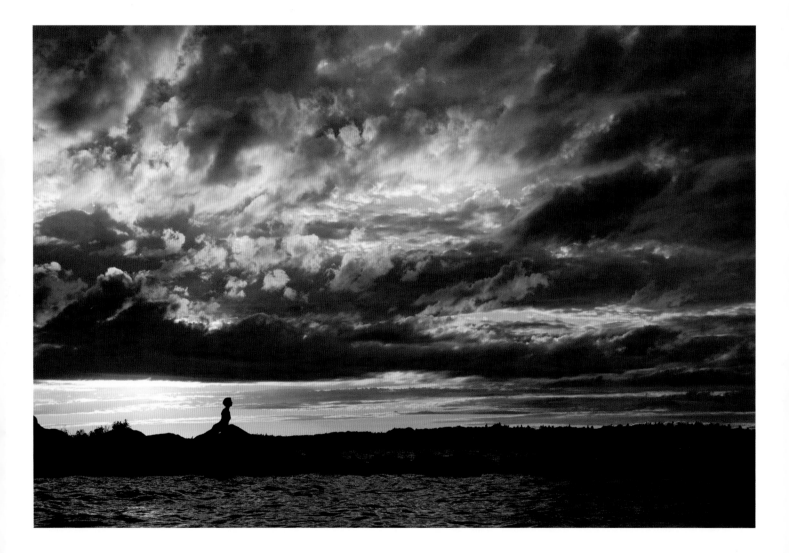

CONFIDENCE

"Do not go where the path may lead, go instead where there is no path and leave a trail."
RALPH WALDO EMERSON

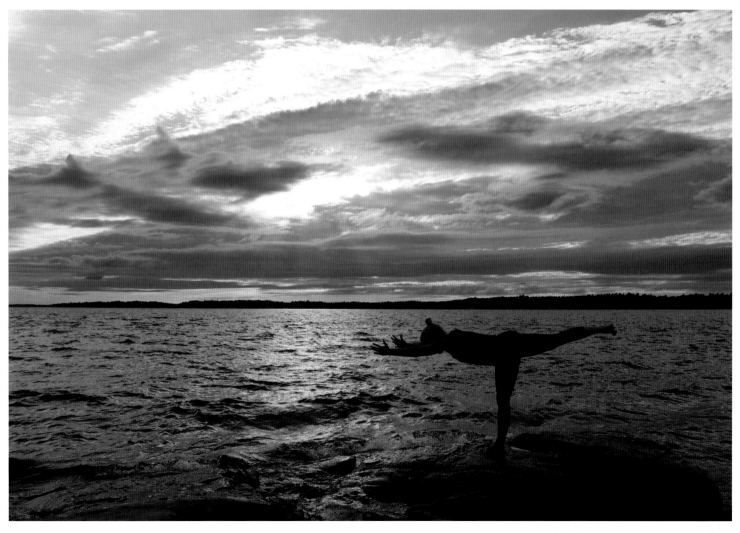

Virabhadrasana III • Warrior Pose Three

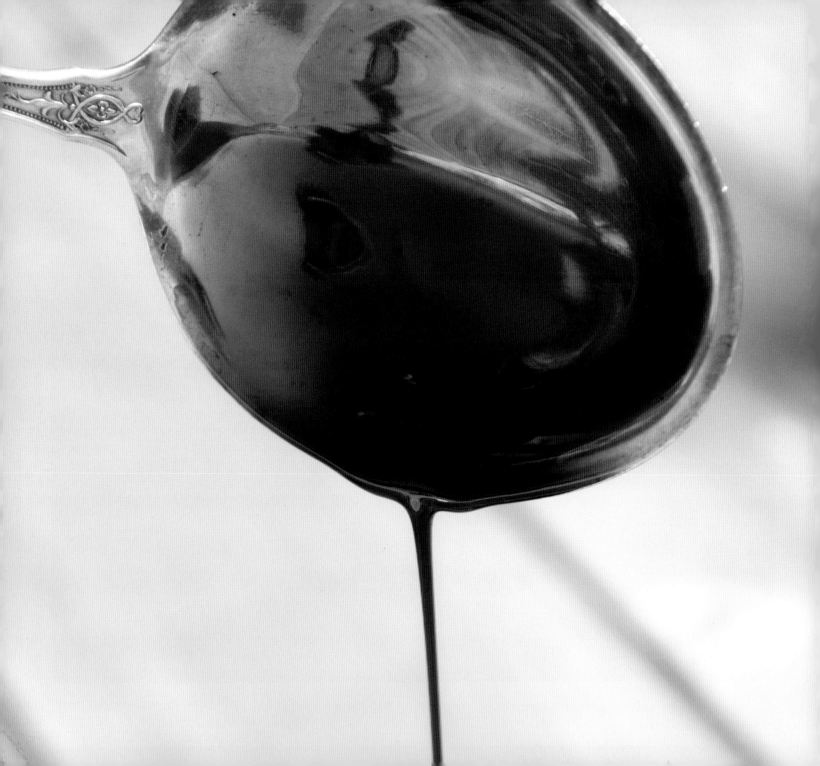

BLAKEY'S BALSAMIC GLAZE (v)

Hummus is a favorite of Liz's daughter, Blake, who once proclaimed, "Hummus is one of the main food groups." Blake will often top a bowl full of hummus with this glaze and eat it with carrots or crackers for dinner. Drizzle it on our So Hum . . . mus (see recipe on page 44) and also Half Moon Hummus Pita (see recipe on page 184). This recipe yields a little less than 1 cup of glaze. It may be stored in the refrigerator for up to 1 week.

    1 cup balsamic vinegar
    ¼ cup brown sugar

1. Place vinegar and brown sugar in small saucepan. Over high heat, bring mixture to a boil.
2. Reduce to a simmer and stir constantly for about 20–30 minutes or until glaze sticks to the back of your stirring spoon.
3. Transfer glaze to a serving dish or container and allow to rest and cool.

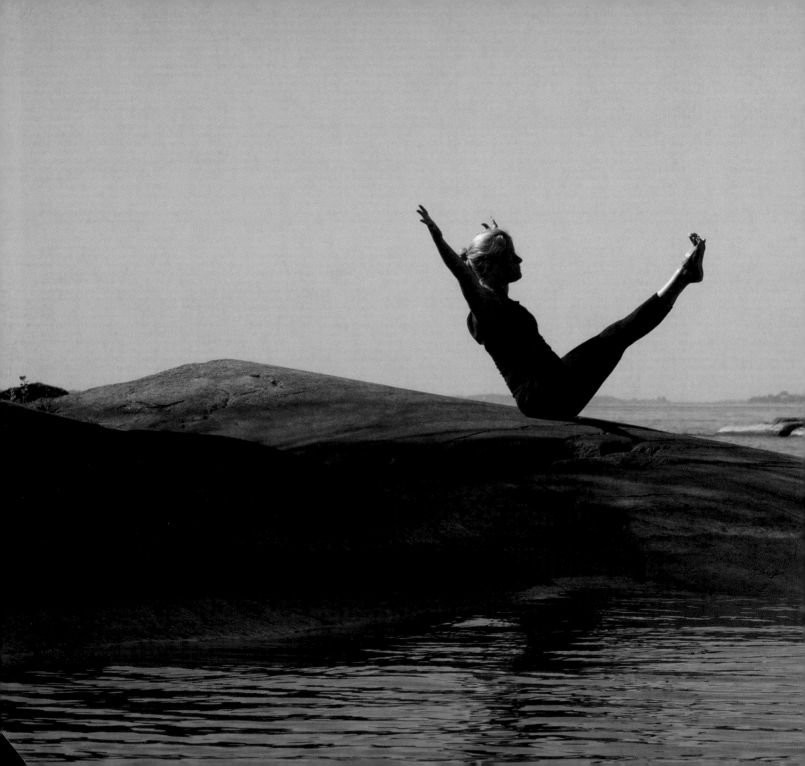

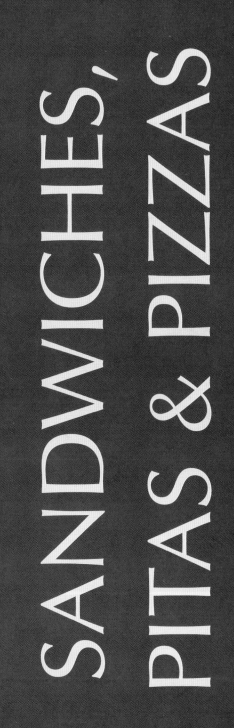

SANDWICHES, PITAS & PIZZAS

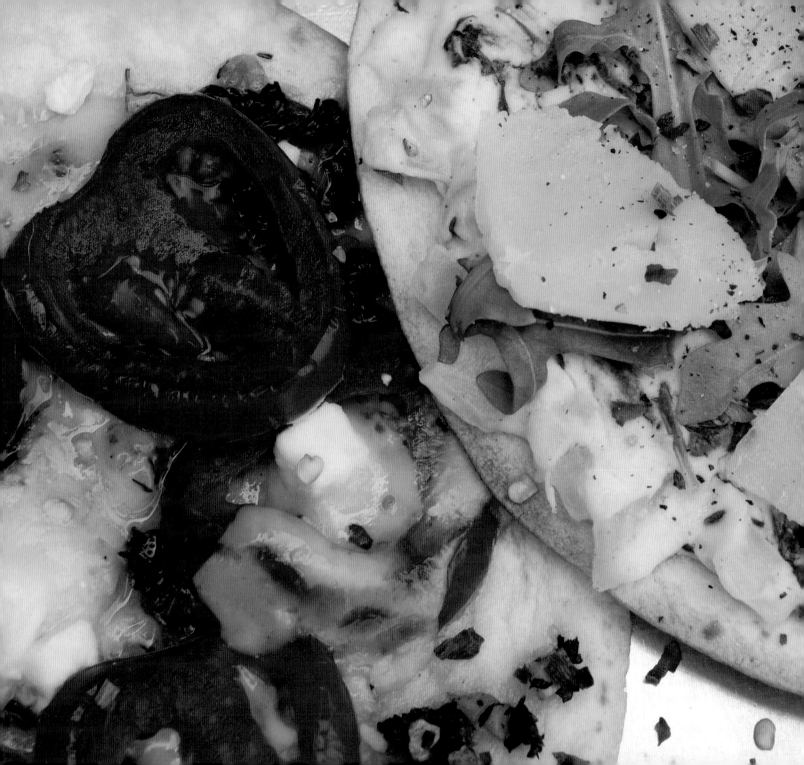

SVELTE PIZZAS

These ultra-thin crust pizzas are light, bold, and decadent. We like to make all three of these recipes and invite friends over for a flavorful and fun pizza party. Variation: Pizzas may be finished on the grill instead of in the oven. Each pizza should serve 2.

TANTILIZING TOASTED HERB
2 medium flour tortillas
2 medium garlic cloves (minced)
1T fresh thyme (chopped)
1T fresh oregano (chopped)
½ cup fresh parsley (chopped)
Himalayan salt coarsely ground (to taste)
Pepper coarsely ground (to taste)

Dash of cayenne pepper
1T olive oil
1 medium tomato (thinly sliced) or *Realized Roasted Tomatoes* (see page 68)
¼ cup feta cheese (crumbled)
¼ cup Gruyere (shredded)
¼ cup fresh Parmesan (shaved)
Hot pepper flakes (optional)

1. Preheat oven to 450°F.
2. Sauté garlic, thyme, oregano, parsley, salt, pepper, and cayenne with olive oil in pan over low-medium heat until garlic and herbs begin to look golden brown or slightly crisped.
3. After garlic and herb mixture is cooked, toast tortillas directly on burners for about 1 minute on each side to start to crisp.
4. Arrange tortillas on lightly greased baking sheet.
5. Top each pizza with half of herb mixture, tomatoes, feta, Gruyere, and Parmesan cheese. Place in preheated oven and bake for about 5–10 minutes or until cheese is melted and edges of tortillas are crisp and golden brown.
6. Remove from oven and garnish each pizza with hot pepper flakes (optional).

AWAKENING ARUGULA
2 medium flour tortillas
2 medium garlic cloves (minced)
½ white onion (chopped)
Himalayan salt coarsely ground (to taste)
Pepper coarsely ground (to taste)
Dash of cayenne pepper
1T olive oil

3 cups arugula (lightly chopped)
½ cup ricotta
¼ cup fresh Parmesan (shaved)
Hot pepper flakes (optional)
Simplicity dressing (see recipe on page 154)

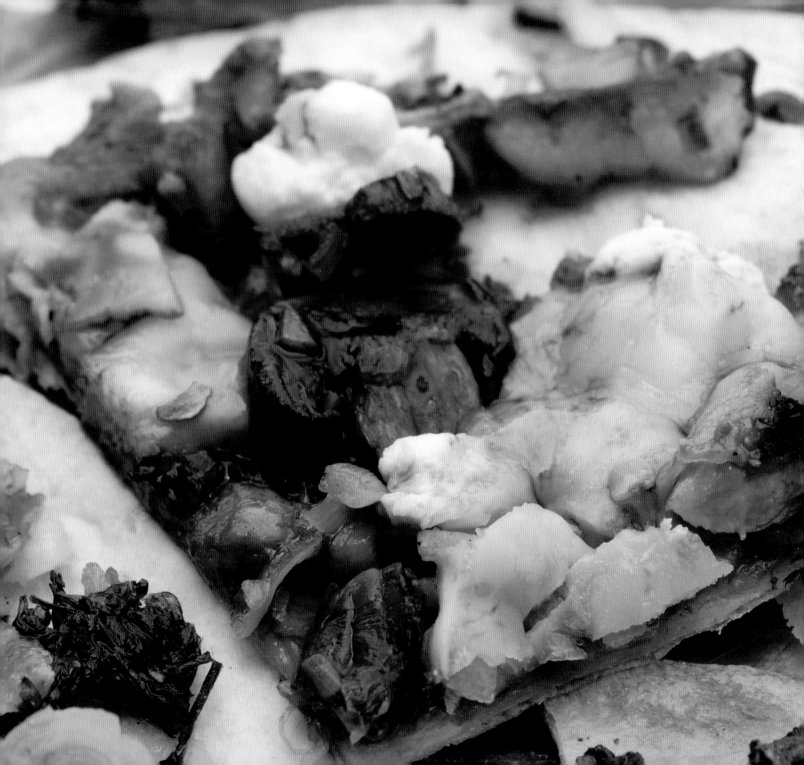

1. Preheat oven to 450°F.
2. Sauté garlic, onion, salt, pepper, and cayenne with olive oil in pan over low-medium heat until garlic and onion soften.
3. Add two cups of arugula and allow to wilt. Remove from heat.
4. Once slightly cooled, add ricotta and combine.
5. After ricotta mixture is prepared, toast tortillas directly on burners for about 1 minute on each side to start to crisp.
6. Arrange tortillas on lightly greased baking sheet.
7. Top each pizza with half of ricotta mixture.
8. Place in preheated oven and bake for about 5–10 minutes or until edges of tortillas are crisp and golden brown.
9. While pizzas are baking, combine remaining cup of arugula with 2 tablespoons of *Simplicity* dressing.
10. Remove pizzas from oven and garnish each pizza with ½ cup of cold arugula salad. Top with shaved Parmesan and hot pepper flakes (optional).

GO WILD MUSHROOM
2 medium flour tortillas
2 medium garlic cloves (minced)
2T shallot (minced)
1 cup wild mushrooms (we like porcini)
2T leeks (chopped)
Himalayan salt coarsely ground (to taste)
Pepper coarsely ground (to taste)
1T olive oil
¼ cup goat cheese (crumbled)
¼ cup fresh Parmesan (shaved)
Hot pepper flakes (optional)
Blakey's Balsamic Glaze (see recipe on page 164)

1. Preheat oven to 450°F.
2. Sauté garlic, shallot, mushrooms, leeks, salt, and pepper with olive oil in pan over low-medium heat until tender.
3. After mushroom mixture is cooked, toast tortillas directly on burners for about 1 minute on each side to start to crisp.
4. Arrange tortillas on lightly greased baking sheet.
5. Top each pizza with half of sautéed mushroom mixture, goat cheese, and Parmesan cheese. Place in preheated oven and bake for about 5–10 minutes or until cheese is melted and edges of tortillas are crisp and golden brown.
6. Remove from oven and garnish each pizza with hot pepper flakes (optional) and about 1 tablespoon of *Blakey's Balsamic Glaze*.

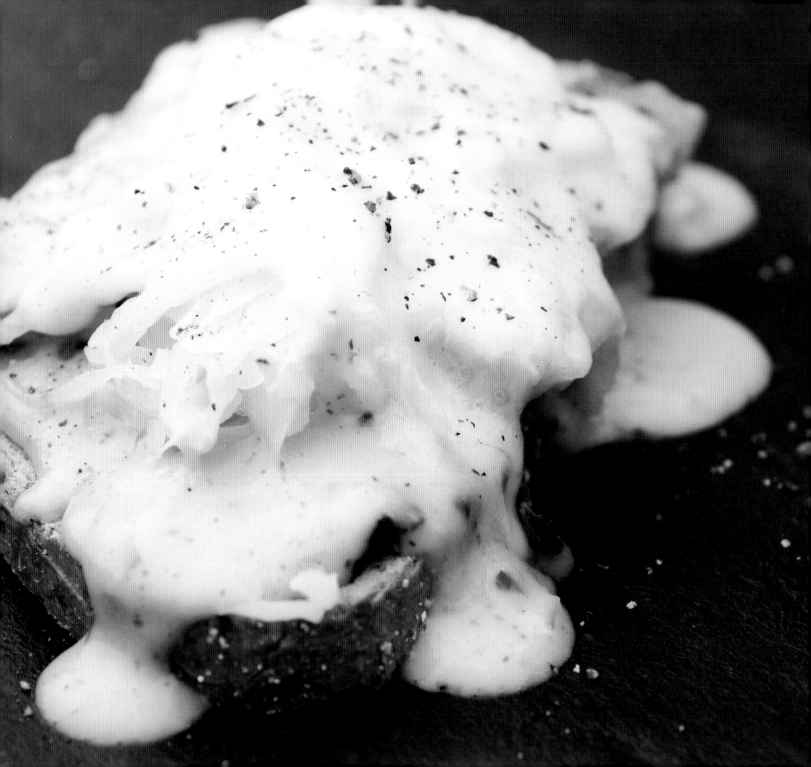

REUBEN REVELATION *(v)*

This tempeh-based Reuben is a healthier alternative to the traditional corned beef Reuben, and we think it's totally robust with flavor and awesome. We use our vegan More than a Thousand Islands dressing for this sandwich. For a completely vegan variation on the sandwich, simply substitute a dairy-free cheese alternative for the Swiss cheese. Serves 4.

Tempeh Marinade
8 oz. tempeh
1T olive oil
½ cup orange juice
¼ tsp. ground ginger
Dash of ground allspice
¼ tsp. mustard seeds
¼ tsp. brown sugar
1T garlic (minced)
Himalayan salt coarsely ground (to taste)
Pepper coarsely ground (to taste)

4 slices Swiss cheese (or vegan alternative)
1 cup fresh sauerkraut
4 large slices rye bread (toasted)

8T *More than a Thousand Islands* dressing (see recipe on page 148)

1. Slice tempeh in half lengthwise to form 2 smaller rectangular pieces. Then slice each piece in half to form 4 thin patties. Combine olive oil, orange juice, ginger, allspice, mustard seeds, sugar, garlic, salt, and pepper to form marinade. Place tempeh in large baking pan and coat all sides of tempeh with marinade. Allow tempeh to rest in marinade for at least 30 minutes before cooking.
2. Place marinated tempeh in medium skillet and begin to sear over medium heat. Cook both sides for about 5 minutes or until crisp and golden brown. Top each slice of tempeh with ¼ of the sauerkraut and 1 slice of cheese. Cover skillet with lid for 1 or 2 minutes to allow cheese to melt and sauerkraut to warm.
3. Toast rye bread. Coat each slice of toast with 1 tablespoon of *More than a Thousand Islands* dressing. Top with tempeh. Serve open face and enjoy!

PARTNER

"Have only love in your heart for others. The more you see the good in them, the more you will establish good in yourself . . . "
PARAMAHANSA YOGANANDA

There is a reason why each and every person is in our lives. Each of our relationships or partnerships—with friends, family, or fellow students—uniquely supports and shapes our growth. We have a responsibility to learn from others and to also share our own inner wisdom.

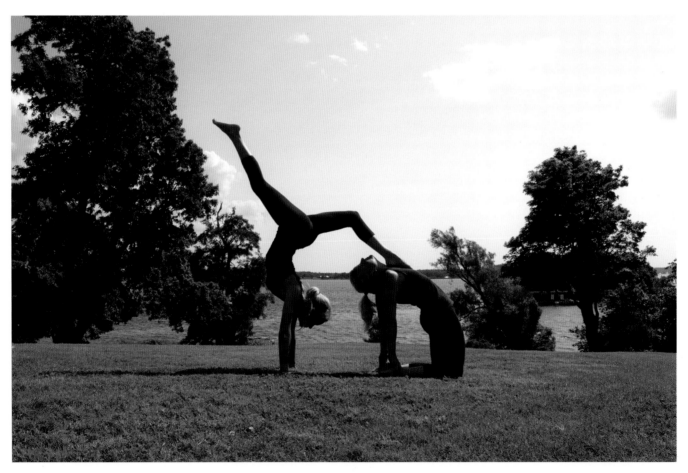

Adho Mukha Vrksasana • Handstand & Ustrasana • Camel Posture

FRIENDSHIP

Find gratitude in friendships. Celebrate friends, family, animals, nature, community, food, and your yoga mat. Authentic friendships are universal, non-harming, and independent of location, age, religion, race, income, gender, *and* time. As with yoga, friendships often take effort, may sometimes be effortless, always offer lessons, and constantly evolve. They are grounded in common experiences and encourage opportunities to grow without bound. Friends often become like family, and true friendships, those indescribable connections of spirit, may impact us on a level beyond our present lives.

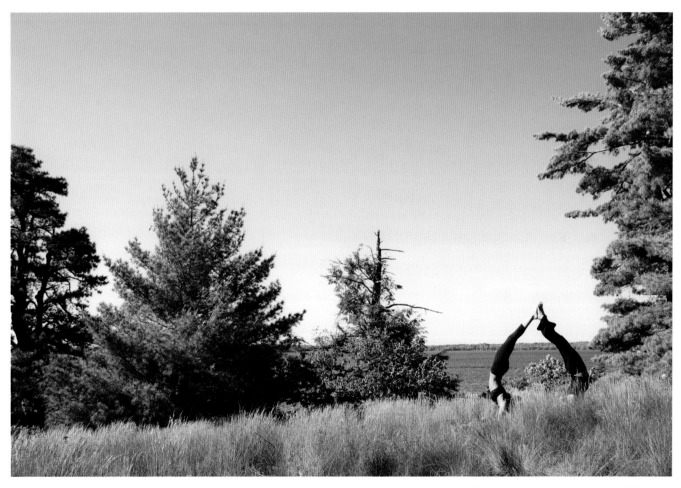

Pincha Mayurasana • Feathered Peacock

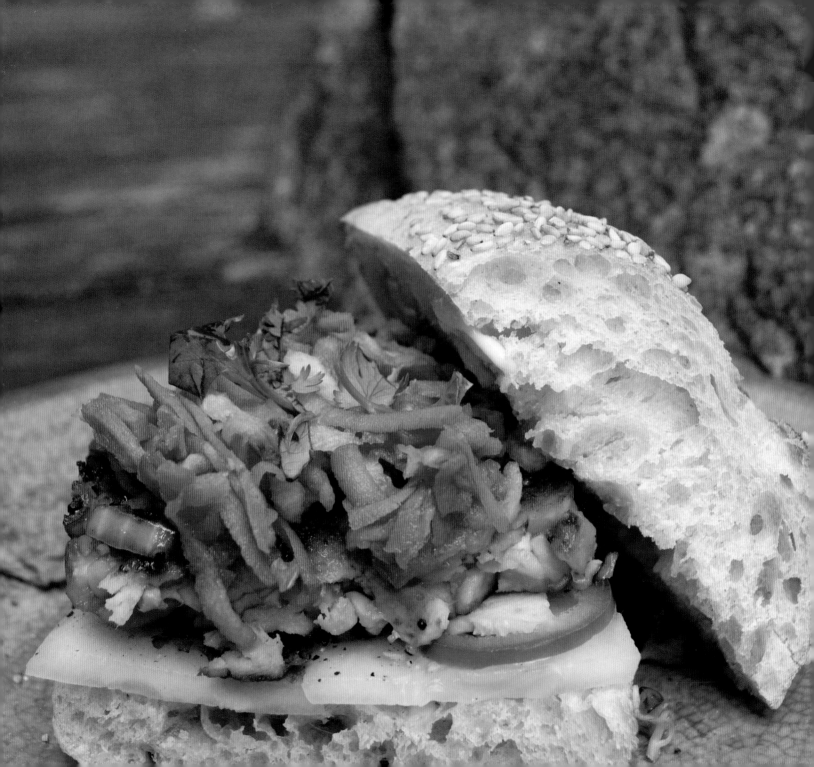

THE HAPPY PIG BANH MI (v)

"Toi muon o banh mi chay." English translation: "I would like a vegan sandwich, please." This is our variation of a classic Vietnamese-style sandwich, "banh mi." Our version is vegan and uses marinated tempeh. The slaw incorporates a traditional Vietnamese dipping sauce, Nuoc Cham, and is also used in our Rice Wheels (see recipe on page 42). Fresh herbs, vegetables, and a crispy baguette finish this sandwich and add to the sandwich's textural and taste-bud-awakening parade. Serves 4.

Marinated Tempeh
8 oz. tempeh
1T olive oil
2T white onion (minced)
2 medium garlic cloves (minced)
1T fresh ginger (minced)
2T tamari
2T orange juice
1T brown sugar
Pepper coarsely ground (to taste)

Slaw
½ cup seasoned rice vinegar
2T tamari
2T lime juice

2 medium garlic cloves (minced)
Red pepper flakes (to taste)
Himalayan salt coarsely ground (to taste)
1 cup carrot (shredded)
1 cup daikon radish (shredded)

1 baguette (large enough for 4 6-inch-long sandwiches)
Vegan mayonnaise (as needed)
½ cup fresh cilantro (chopped)
8 slices cucumber (cut lengthwise)
Pepper coarsely ground (to taste)
2 jalapeños, sliced with seeds (optional)
Scallions, chopped (optional)

1. Preheat oven to 400°F.
2. Slice tempeh in half lengthwise to form 2 smaller rectangular pieces. Then slice each piece in half to form 4 thin patties. Combine olive oil, onion, garlic, ginger, tamari, orange juice, sugar, and pepper to form marinade. Place tempeh in large baking pan and coat all sides of tempeh with marinade. Allow tempeh to rest in marinade for at least 30 minutes before cooking.
3. Combine rice vinegar, tamari, lime juice, garlic, red pepper flakes, and salt in a medium mixing bowl to create slaw dressing. Once combined, mix in shredded carrot and daikon. Set aside.
4. Place marinated tempeh in medium skillet and begin to sear over medium heat. Cook both sides for about 5 minutes or until crisp and golden brown. Cover in foil to keep warm.
5. Slice baguettes in half lengthwise to form a sandwich vessel and then cut into 4 6-inch sandwich buns. Coat the insides of the baguettes with vegan mayonnaise. Place baguettes on baking sheet and bake until hot and crispy or for about 5 minutes.
6. On each toasted bun, layer slices of cucumber, chopped cilantro, ground pepper, jalapeños, scallions, a cooked tempeh patty, and slaw. Close the sandwiches. Serve and enjoy immediately.

VEGETARIANISM

"The doctor of the future will give no medication, but will interest his patients in the care of the human frame, diet and in the cause and prevention of disease."
THOMAS A. EDISON

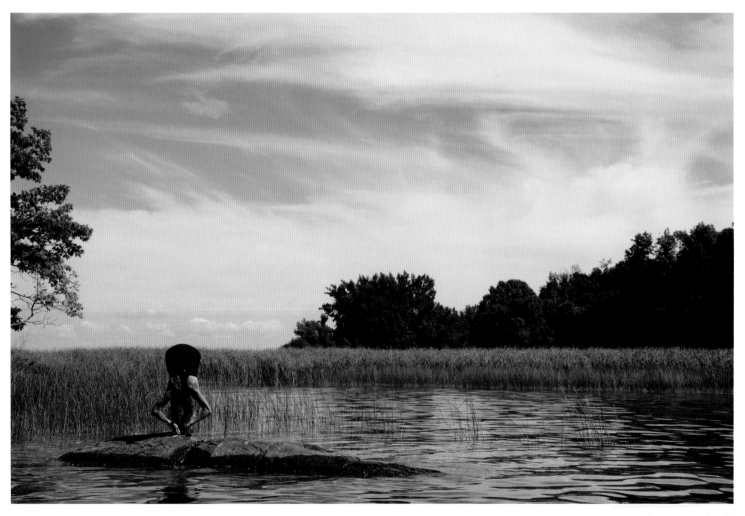

Uttanasana I • Standing Forward Fold

MINDFULNESS

"Your body is precious. It is our vehicle for awakening. Treat it with care."
GAUTAMA BUDDHA

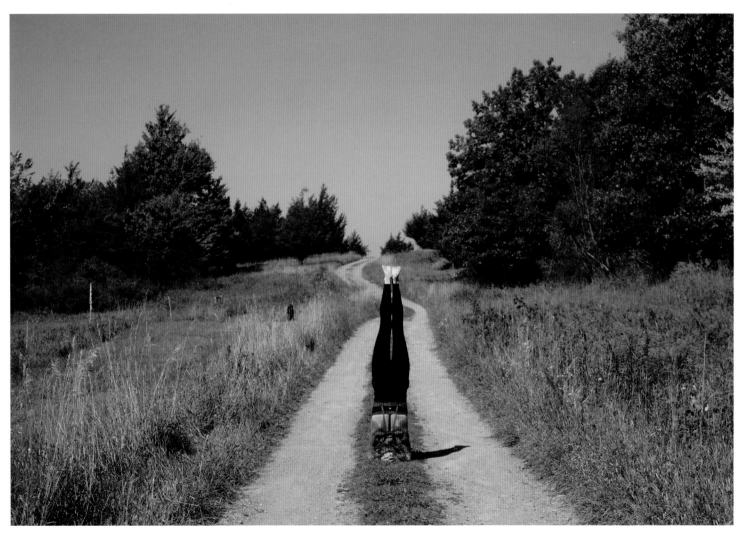

Salamba Sirsasana • Supported Headstand

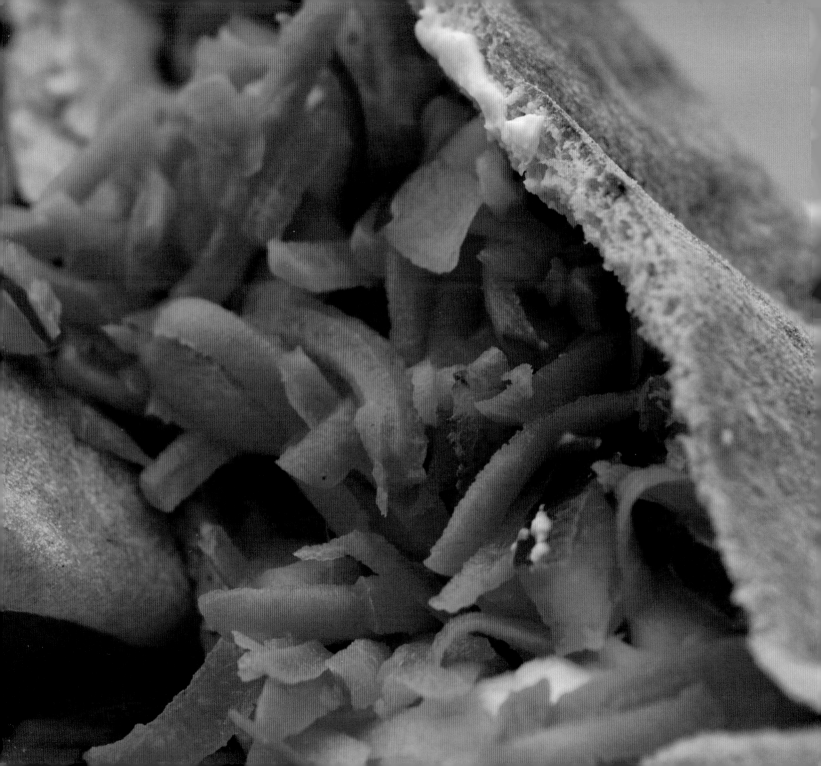

RADIANT CARROT SALAD PITA *(v)*

This recipe utilizes our energizing Radiant Carrots. Nutritional yeast is a deactivated yeast that is packed with vitamins and protein. An easy and joyful pita recipe, this may be topped with organic alfalfa sprouts as well. Serves 4.

Radiant Carrots (see recipe on page 78)

4 oz. cream cheese (or cream cheese substitute)
2T nutritional yeast
4 medium pitas (halved)

1. Prepare *Radiant Carrots* recipe (prepare a half recipe if just using carrots for sandwiches or a whole recipe if you'd like some yummy leftovers!).
2. In a small bowl, mix together cream cheese and nutritional yeast.
3. Spread cream cheese and nutritional yeast mixture equally between 8 pita halves.
4. Add equal amounts of *Radiant Carrots* to each pita half.
5. Serve each person 2 pita halves.

HOME

"The purpose of all major religious traditions is not to construct big temples on the outside, but to create temples of goodness and compassion inside, in our hearts."
DALAI LAMA

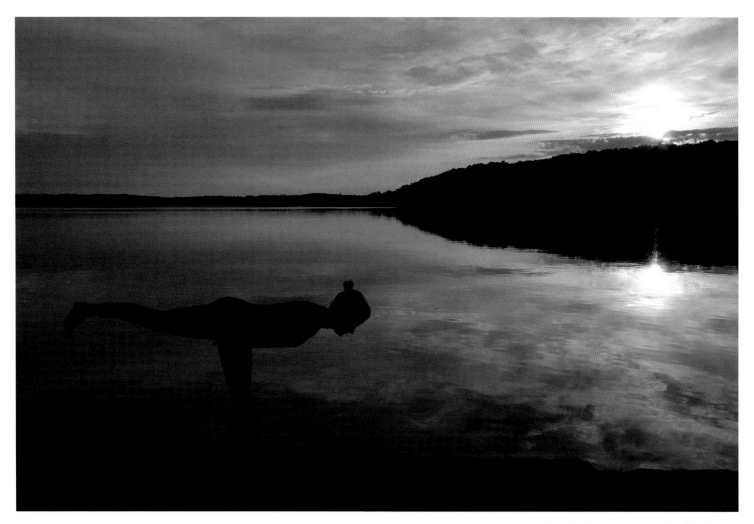

Virabhadrasana III • Warrior Pose Three

ARDHA CHANDRASANA I
HALF MOON POSE

*balancing, reduces emotional fatigue, improves digestion,
increases focus and concentration*

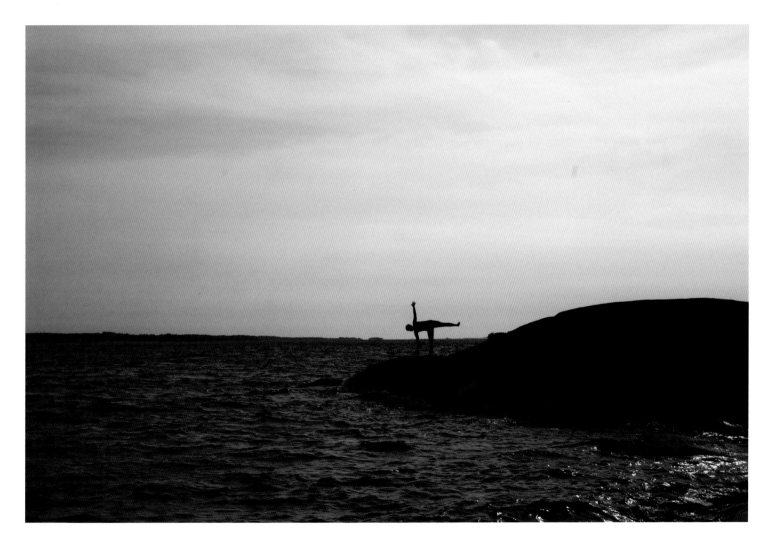

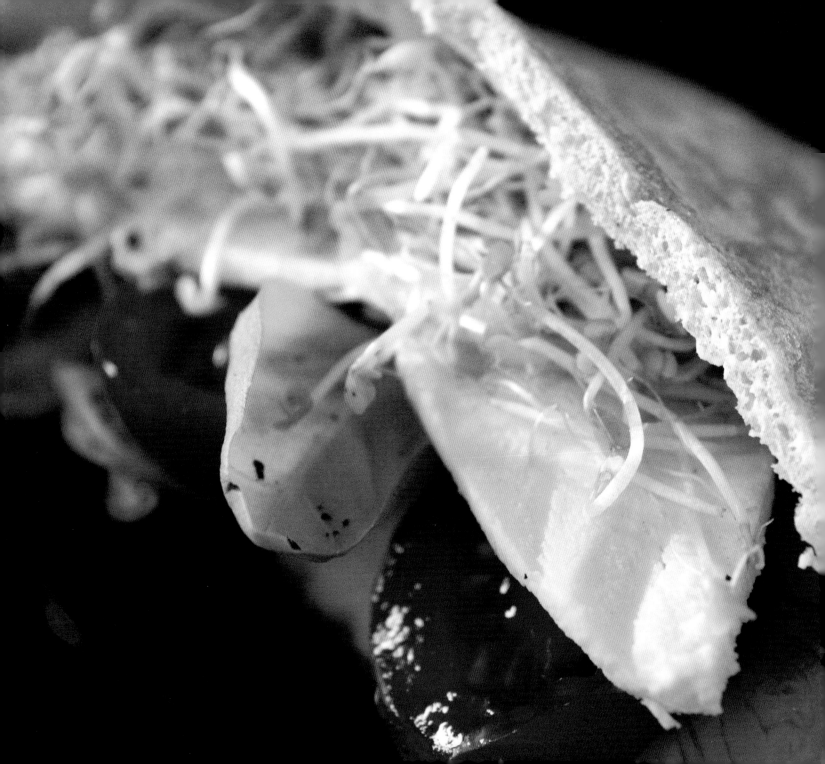

HALF MOON PITA HUMMUS *(v)*

In yoga, the sun and the moon are symbolically powerful, representing polar energies of the body. Many yoga postures, such as Half Moon Pose (see previous page) were designed to help us stretch in opposing directions from limb to limb. This helps us to restore balance in the body. With balance, we are able to conduct our lives at just the right place— between effort and ease. Our Half Moon Hummus Pita pairs with our So Hum . . . mus. It provides a balance of flavors and is also, appropriately, served in half-pitas, the shape of half moons. Serves 4.

So Hum . . . mus (see recipe on page 44)

4 medium pitas (halved)
1 medium shallot (minced)
½ cup fresh basil (chopped)
1 medium cucumber (sliced into rounds)
1 cup fresh sprouts
1 medium tomato (thinly sliced)
8 oz. thinly sliced fresh mozzarella (optional)
Himalayan salt coarsely ground (to taste)
Pepper coarsely ground (to taste)

1. Prepare *So Hum . . . mus* recipe (prepare a half recipe if just using hummus for sandwiches or a whole recipe if you'd like some yummy leftovers!).
2. In each pita half equally spread each of the following ingredients: shallot, basil, cucumber, sprouts, tomato, mozzarella, and salt and pepper to taste.
3. Serve immediately and enjoy!

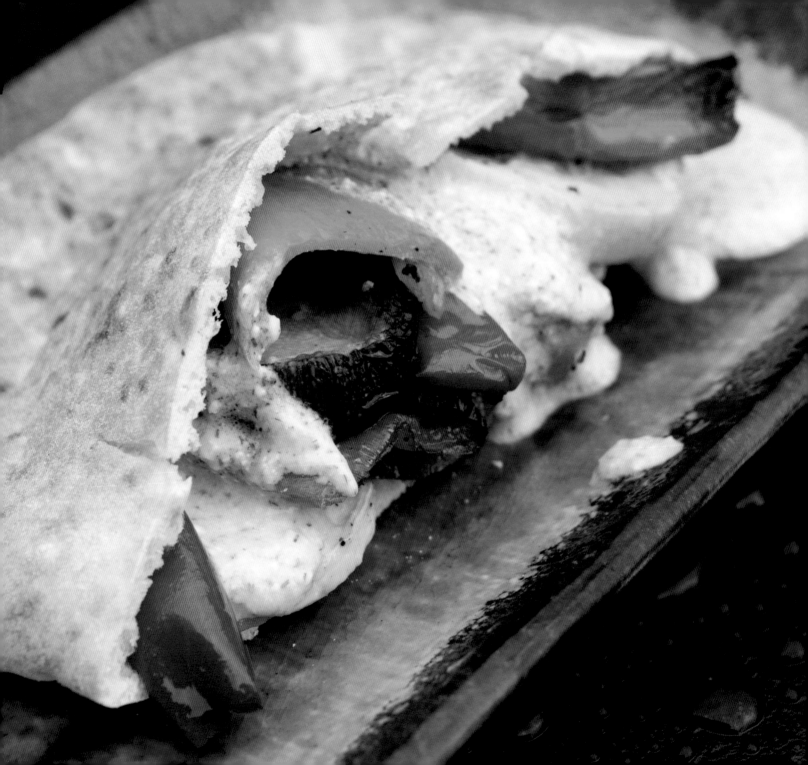

ADVENTUROUS VEGETABLE

When following ahimsa (non-harming), we are mindful of our bodies' needs. Sometimes, that means going on an adventure or taking our practices to a place we did not know existed before. This dish is warm and hearty. Please feel free to substitute the vegetables based on what you enjoy. Serves 8.

Herbed Feta Spread
8 oz. feta (crumbled)
3T water
2T olive oil
2T lemon juice
½ cup parsley (chopped)
½ cup mint (chopped)
½ cup basil (chopped)
½ cup dill (chopped)

3T olive oil
4 large garlic cloves (minced)

1 large eggplant (peeled, salted and rinsed, and cut into slices)
2 green squash (sliced)
2 yellow squash (sliced)
1 large white onion (sliced)
20 small multi-colored sweet peppers (de-ribbed, seeded, and quartered)
Himalayan salt coarsely ground (to taste)
Pepper coarsely ground (to taste)

8 pitas (toasted)

1. Preheat oven to 350°F.
2. Make *Herbed Feta Spread*. Combine feta, water, and olive oil in a food processor. Once smooth, add lemon juice and herbs and process just to combine. Set aside.
3. Combine garlic and vegetables with olive oil and salt and pepper to taste. Pour onto baking sheet in an even layer. Bake for about 30 minutes or until vegetables are slightly browned and fork tender.
4. Remove vegetables from oven and toast pitas by placing halved pitas on baking sheets and toasting them in the oven for about 1 minute on each side.
5. Assemble pitas. Place about 2 tablespoons of *Herbed Feta Spread* in each toasted pita half. Distribute roasted vegetables equally among pita halves (about ½ cup in each pita half).
6. Serve and enjoy immediately.

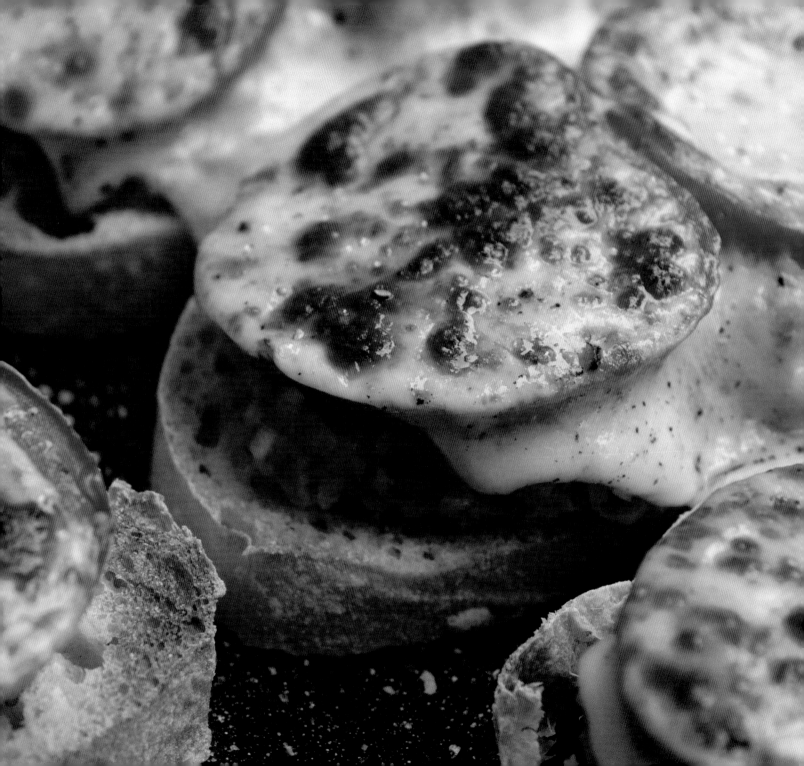

THOUGHTFUL NOT-TOO-TUNA MELT (v)

"Never doubt that a small group of thoughtful, committed citizens can change the world. Indeed, it is the only thing that ever has." MARGARET MEAD

Our Thoughtful Not-Too-Tuna Melt follows the guidelines of non-harming (ahimsa), as the chickpea and nut base of this dish is vegan. It is packed with flavor, and the melt provides that sandwich satisfaction that we all crave from time to time. Serves 4.

15 oz. canned chickpeas
1 cup raw walnuts (soaked in water for 1 hour)
½ cup celery (chopped)
½ cup bread and butter–style pickles (chopped)
¼ cup red onions (minced)
3T dill (chopped)
2T agave nectar
3T lemon juice
2T Dijon mustard
1T vegan mayonnaise
Dash of cayenne pepper
Himalayan salt coarsely ground (to taste)
Pepper coarsely ground (to taste)

4 slices bread
1 pear (thinly sliced) or 1 tomato (thinly sliced)
4 slices cheese (or vegan alternative)

1. Coarsely chop drained and rinsed chickpeas and drained walnuts in a food processor.
2. In a medium mixing bowl, combine chickpeas and walnuts with celery, pickles, onion, dill, agave, lemon, mustard, mayonnaise, cayenne, salt, and pepper. Set aside.
3. Toast bread.
4. Top each piece of toast with ¼ of the *Thoughtful Not-Too-Tuna* mixture and then slices of pear or tomato. Top with cheese of choice.
5. Place open-faced sandwiches on a baking sheet and broil until cheese is bubbly and starting to look golden brown.
6. Remove from oven and serve.

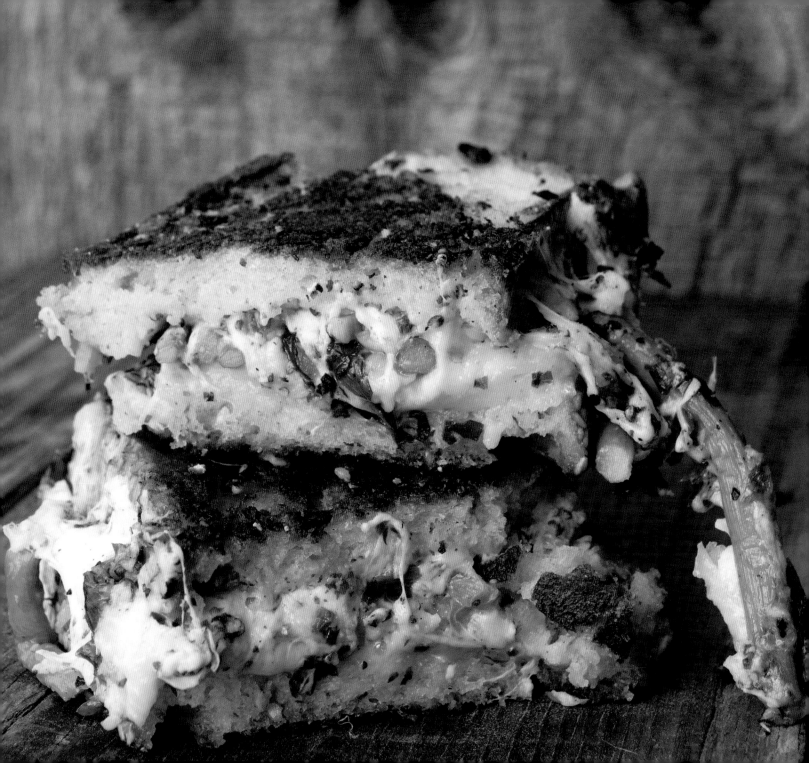

ASPARAGUS ASHRAM

"Breath is the gateway to our inner landscapes." LIZ PRICE-KELLOGG

An Ashram is a spiritual monastery or place which often offers cultural teachings of yoga, spiritual practices, or religion. These teachings help us to continue to develop our awareness and guide us on our paths to our best selves.

Our Asparagus Ashram sandwich is a veggie-packed but still decadent grilled cheese sandwich. Create and savor. Serves 4.

3T olive oil
2 medium garlic cloves (minced)
1T shallot (minced)
20 thin asparagus spears (large stems removed)
Himalayan salt coarsely ground (to taste)
Pepper coarsely ground (to taste)
1T lemon juice
2T fresh basil (chopped)

1T flat leaf parsley (chopped)
Dash of cayenne pepper
1 cup grated sharp cheddar cheese (we use River Rat XXX Sharp)
½ cup grated smoked Gouda cheese
8 oz. thinly sliced mozzarella cheese
8 slices good bread
4T grainy French mustard

1. In a large skillet over medium heat, sauté garlic, shallot, and asparagus with salt and pepper to taste with 1 tablespoon of olive oil until asparagus is tender, or for about 10 minutes.
2. Turn off heat and add lemon juice, basil, parsley, and cayenne. Combine. Use a spatula to remove asparagus mixture from skillet and set aside in a bowl.
3. Mix cheddar and Gouda cheeses together in a medium mixing bowl.
4. Place cheddar and Gouda mixture, equally, on 4 slices of the bread. Add equal amounts of asparagus mixture onto each piece of bread with grated cheese. Top with sliced mozzarella equally on each sandwich half. Spread 1 tablespoon of mustard on the inside of each top bread slice. Place one slice of bread on top of each sandwich half.
5. In the same skillet used to cook asparagus, heat 1 tablespoon of olive oil over medium heat. Add sandwiches to skillet and brush top bread slices with remaining 1 tablespoon of olive oil.
6. Place a lid over the skillet and cook the sandwiches for about 5 minutes on each side or until bread is golden brown and cheese is melted.
7. Cut sandwiches in half (if desired) and serve immediately.

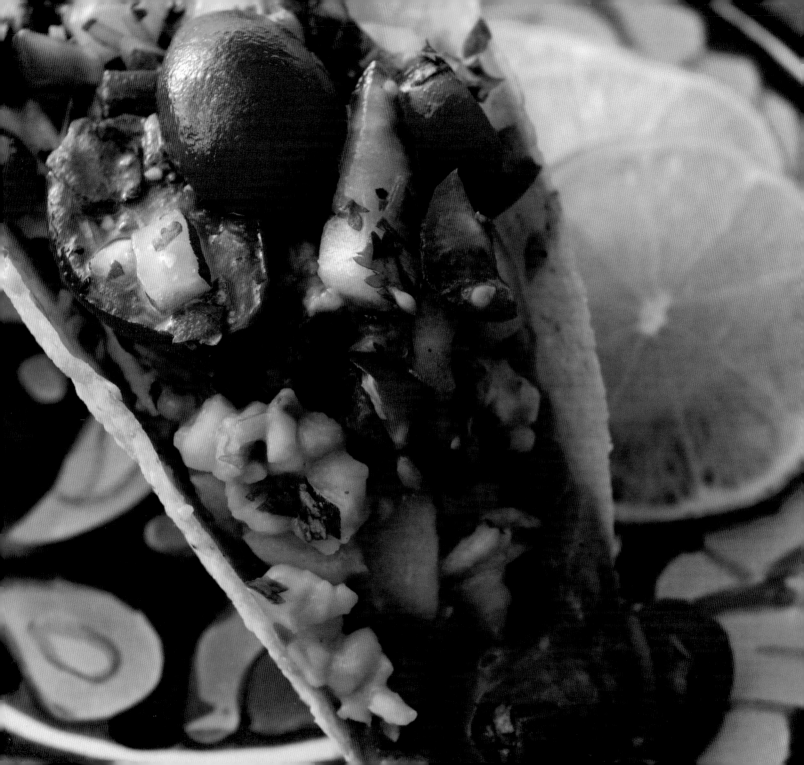

TWISTED TACOS (v)

In twisting postures, we are able to shift our perspectives, detoxify, and gather new insight and strength. Our Twisted Tacos are layered with flavor and the ingredients provide great protein and nutrition. Serves 8.

Fresh Salsa
1 cup cherry tomatoes (diced)
¼ red onion (diced)
1 medium garlic clove (minced)
½ jalapeño (seeded, de-ribbed, and minced)
¼ cup cilantro (chopped)
1T lime juice
Himalayan salt coarsely ground (to taste)
Pepper coarsely ground (to taste)
1T olive oil

Holy Guacamole (see recipe on page 44)

Refined Beans
1T olive oil
1 medium garlic clove (minced)
½ medium white onion (minced)
1 tsp. chili powder
Dash of cayenne pepper
¼ tsp. ground cumin
Himalayan salt coarsely ground (to taste)
Pepper coarsely ground (to taste)
15 oz. pinto beans (drained and rinsed)
1 cup vegetable broth

8 taco shells of choice (we prefer hard taco shells for the crunch)

1. Preheat oven to 300°F.
2. Prepare *Fresh Salsa* by combining all ingredients.
3. Prepare *Holy Guacamole* recipe.
4. Prepare *Refined Beans* by heating oil in a medium skillet over low-medium heat. Add garlic and onion and sauté for 5 minutes. Add spices, beans, and broth. Cook for about 10 minutes, mashing beans with a spoon, spatula, or potato masher and fully combining with broth. Remove from heat.
5. Place tacos on an ungreased baking sheet. Place in oven for 5 minutes to warm.
6. Assemble tacos. Place 3 tablespoons of beans in warmed taco. Top with 2 tablespoons of *Holy Guacamole* and then 2 tablespoons of *Fresh Salsa*.
7. Serve immediately and enjoy!

PARIVRTTA TRIKONASANA
REVOLVED TRIANGLE POSE

detoxifying, relaxes nervous system, releases tension

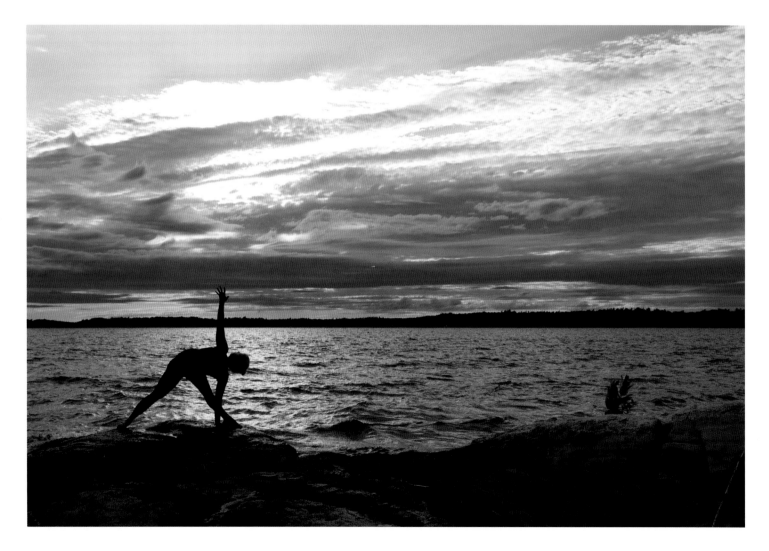

FLEXIBILITY

"The strength of a tree lies in its ability to bend."
ZEN PROVERB

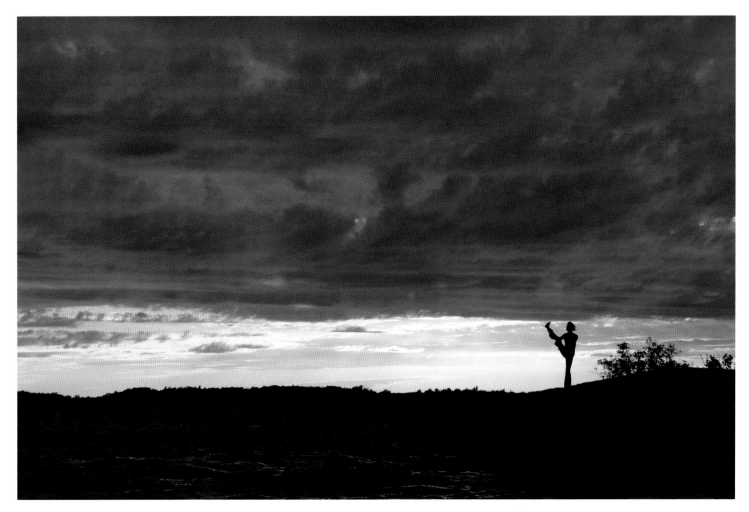

Svarga Dvijasana • Bird of Paradise

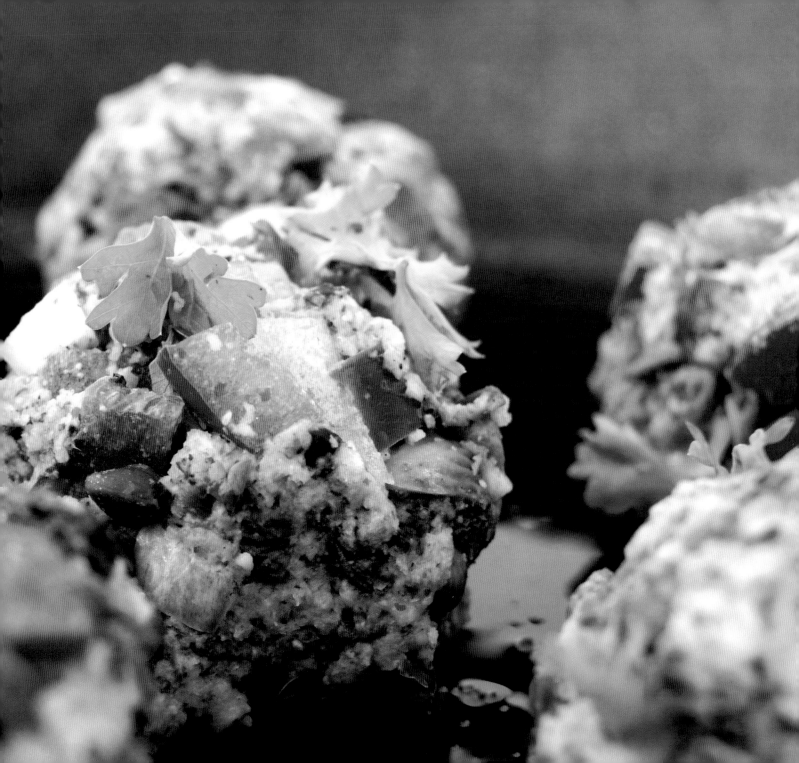

BOUNTIFUL BURGER (v)

Not all veggie burgers are made equal. . . This is a world-class burger packed with fiber and flavor, providing total satisfaction for body and mind. Variation: Serve burgers in sandwich buns. Our Bountiful Burger is also completely delicious when topped with Dijon mustard or our Vegan Green Goddess dressing (see recipe on page 148). Serves 4.

1 cup dried wild mushrooms (reconstituted)
½ cup walnuts (chopped and toasted)
1 red bell pepper (diced)
2T tamari
1T capers
1 medium shallot (minced)
4 medium garlic cloves (minced)
2T Dijon mustard
½ cup seasoned breadcrumbs

2T fresh parsley (chopped)
1T fresh thyme (chopped)
2T chickpea flour, wheat flour, or ground flax seeds
Dash of cayenne pepper
Himalayan salt coarsely ground (to taste)
Pepper coarsely ground (to taste)
1T olive oil
1 cup fresh arugula
1T lemon juice

1. Reconstitute dried mushrooms per package instructions and then drain and chop. Set aside.
2. Toast nuts in a medium skillet over low-medium heat, adding salt to taste throughout the process, until golden brown and fragrant. Remove from heat and set aside.
3. In a medium mixing bowl, combine mushrooms, walnuts, red bell pepper, tamari, capers, shallot, garlic, Dijon, breadcrumbs, parsley, thyme, flour or flax seeds, cayenne, and salt and pepper to taste.
4. Take half of the burger mixture and place it in a food processor. Pulse the mixture a few times and then recombine with the remaining burger ingredients. (This will help the burgers to hold their shape while cooking.)
5. Using your hands, divide the mixture into quadrants. Form each quadrant into a round patty.
6. Pour olive oil in skillet over medium heat. Place patties in skillet and sear for about 5 minutes on each side or until the outside of the burgers are crisped.
7. While burgers are cooking, combine arugula, lemon juice, and salt and pepper to taste in a small mixing bowl.
8. Arrange burgers on beds of dressed arugula and serve.

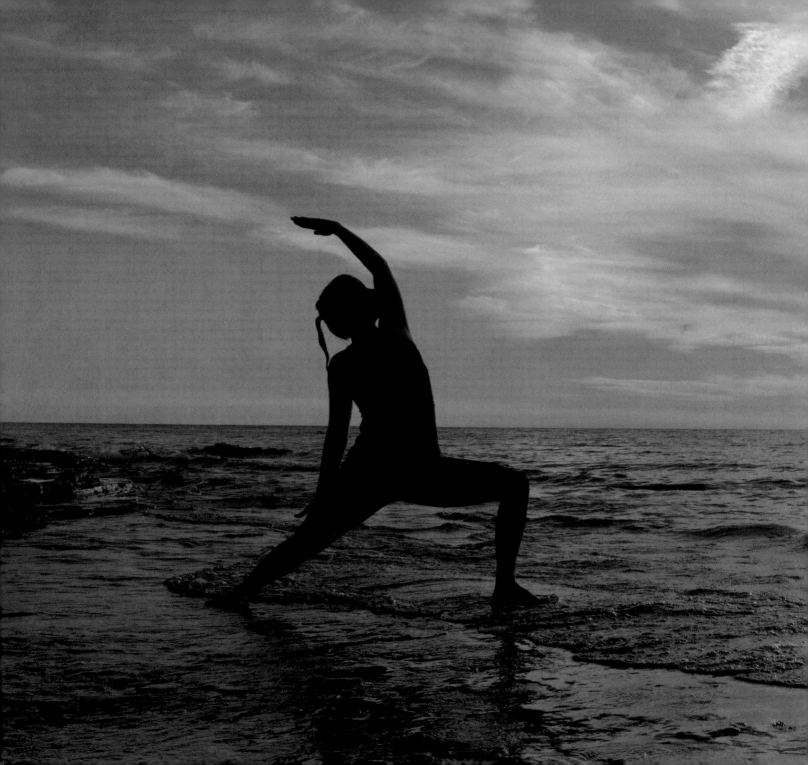

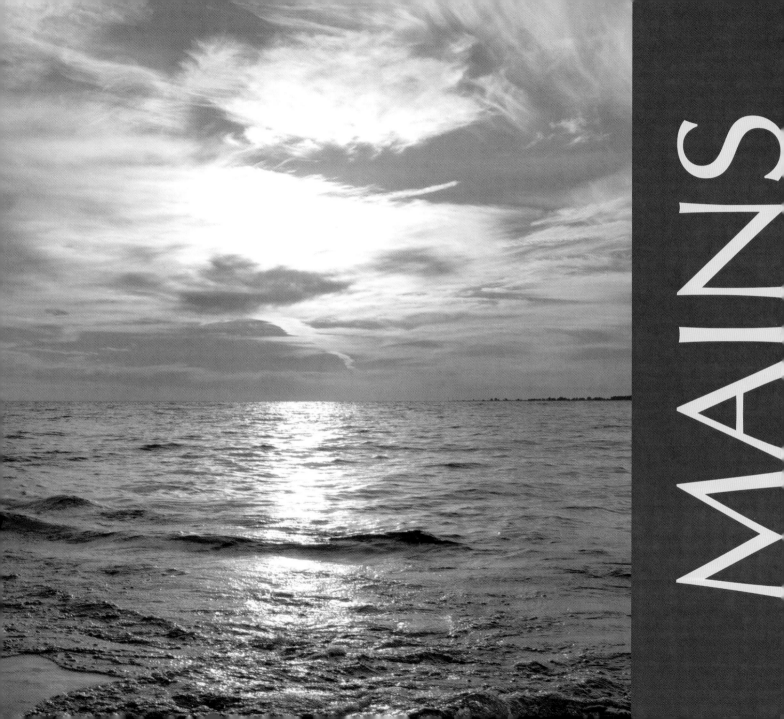

MAINS

ACTION

*"As we express our gratitude, we must never forget that the highest appreciation
is not to utter words, but to live by them."*
JOHN F. KENNEDY

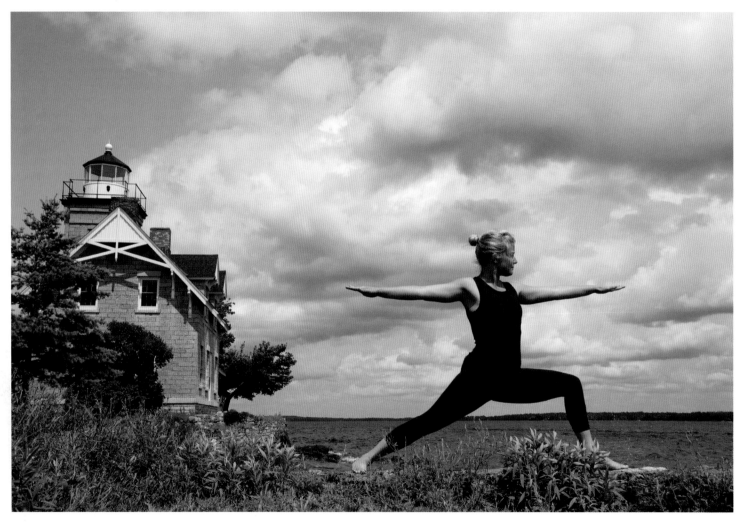

Virabhadrasana II • Warrior Pose Two

VIPARITA VIRABHADRASANA
EXALTED WARRIOR POSE

dynamic, teaches presence, increases agility and strength

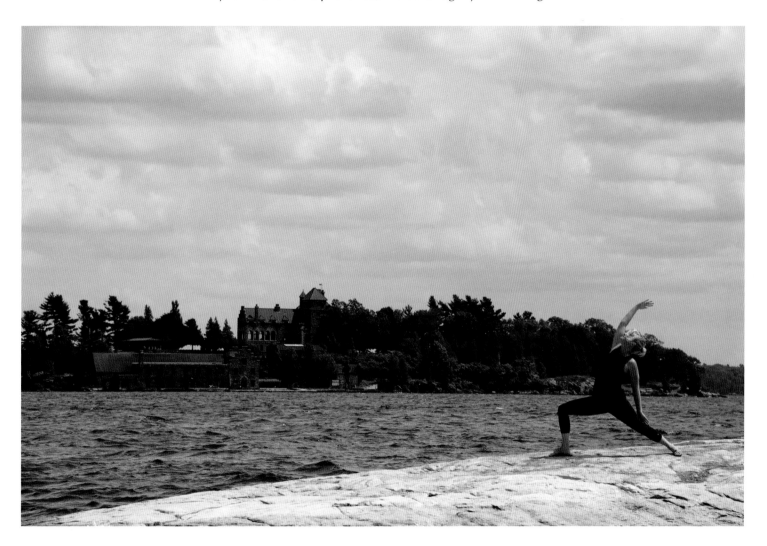

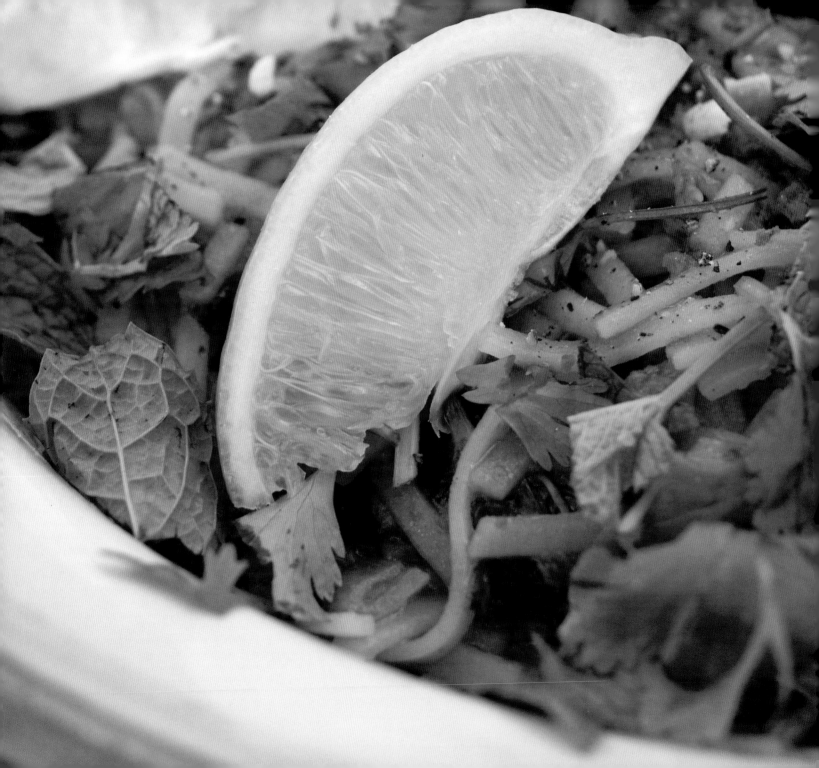

WARRIOR NOODLES *(v)*

When we think of yogis, we typically think of peaceful, thoughtful, mindful individuals. Thus creating the question, "Why warrior?" Virabhadra is a warrior in the Hindu religion and Warrior Poses (Virabhadrasana) carry his namesake. Warrior 1 Pose is a difficult posture that requires flexibility and strength of the body and mind. Often, Warrior 1 Pose makes us feel uncomfortable, revealing to us where we may need to dig deeper or let go. Importantly, we all have a warrior within us that may help us to battle or overcome issues with ego, ignorance, or ill will. Our Warrior Noodles is a Thai-inspired dish designed to embolden. Serves 4–6.

No-Fish Fish Sauce
4T tamari
6T rice vinegar
6T water
3T agave
3T (heaping) Asian chili garlic sauce
1T Asian hot sauce or to taste

10 oz. Asian noodles (Udon or Rice)
3 large garlic cloves (diced)

3 medium shallots (cut in half lengthwise and then sliced)
2T olive oil
12 oz. vegetable protein crumbles (variation: use 2 cups fresh broccoli)
1 cup (loosely packed) cilantro (lightly chopped)
1 cup (loosely packed) mint (lightly chopped)
½ cup salted peanuts (coarsely chopped or pounded with back of wooden spoon in plastic bag; variation: use salted cashews)
1 lime (cut into wedges for serving)

1. Prepare *No-Fish Fish Sauce*.
2. Start preparing noodles per package instructions or cook until al dente.
3. Over medium-low heat in a large skillet, sauté garlic and shallot with olive oil until just tender.
4. Add *No-Fish Fish Sauce* to skillet. Simmer for 1 minute.
5. Turn heat to low and add veggie crumbles (if substituting broccoli, cook in pasta water before or after pasta until just tender, then combine into skillet mix at this point).
6. Add cooked pasta, ½ of the cilantro, and ½ of the mint. Combine.
7. Plate and serve immediately, topping noodles with remaining cilantro, mint, and nuts. Serve lime wedges on the side. Enjoy!

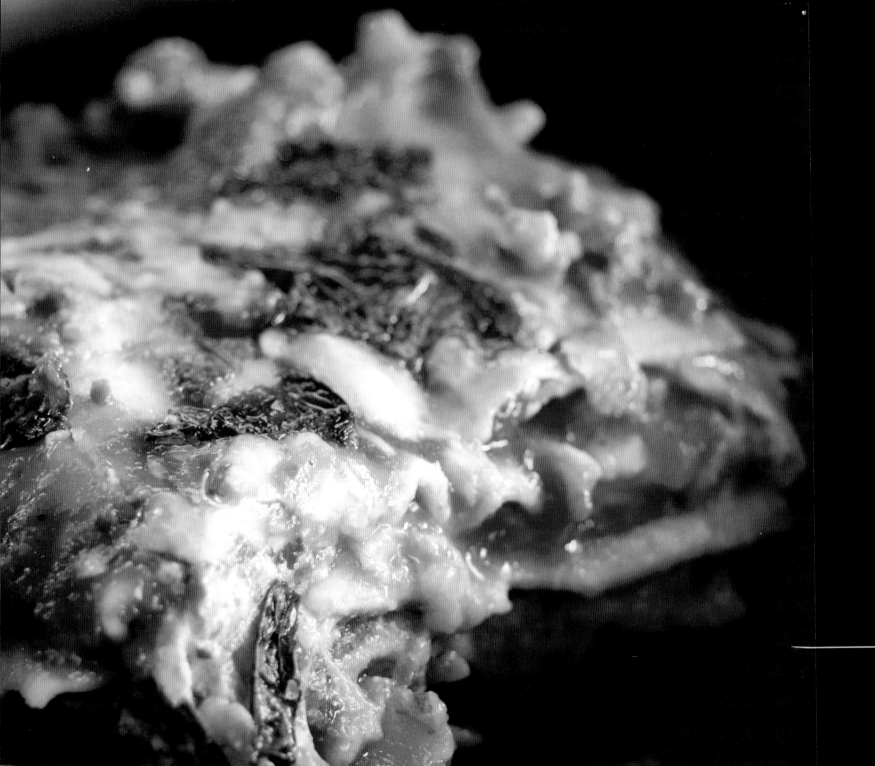

LOTUS "LIZ"AGNA

"Life is a combination of magic and pasta." FEDERICO FELLINI

This is a dish that Liz has been serving to grateful friends and family for years, and according to Kristen's carnivorous husband, it is so delicious that "it doesn't even need meat." Comforting, grounding, simple, and satiating, it is the perfect entrée for large parties and also makes for excellent leftovers. You may use our Prana Pesto (see recipe on page 46) and Pleasant Peasant Tomato Sauce (see recipe on page 222) to prepare this dish. If you choose to buy premade sauces, choose quality, local products. This dish pairs wonderfully with our Karma Kale salad with Cobra Caesar dressing. Serves 12–16.

1 large white onion (diced)
5 garlic cloves (diced)
Dash of cayenne pepper
8 oz. pesto
4–5 cups organic fresh spinach or kale
16 oz. cottage cheese
16 oz. ricotta

2 eggs
24 oz. marinara sauce
12 oz. lasagna noodles
2 8 oz. balls of mozzarella (sliced plus some for top)
1 cup fresh basil (chopped)

1. Preheat oven to 375°F.
2. Sauté onion and garlic until tender. Add dash of cayenne pepper.
3. Add pesto and spinach or kale. Combine until greens wilt.
4. Remove mixture from heat and allow to cool to room temperature. Once the mixture is cool add cottage cheese, ricotta, and eggs. Combine.
5. In a 13 x 9 inch baking dish, begin layering lasagna, starting with the marinara sauce. Next add a layer of uncooked lasagna noodles, followed by the ricotta mixture and then a layer of the sliced mozzarella. Continue the layering process until you nearly reach the top of the baking dish. Then add a last thin layer of marinara sauce. Grate any remaining mozzarella cheese and sprinkle on top.
6. Place the dish in the oven and bake with aluminum foil for about 35 minutes or until bubbling. Remove the foil and bake for an additional 10 minutes or until the top of the lasagna is slightly golden brown.
7. Remove the lasagna from the oven and top with fresh basil.
8. Allow it to set in the dish for at least 10 minutes. Slice, serve, and enjoy.

PADMASANA
LOTUS POSTURE

grounding, calming, meditative, increases flexibility in hips

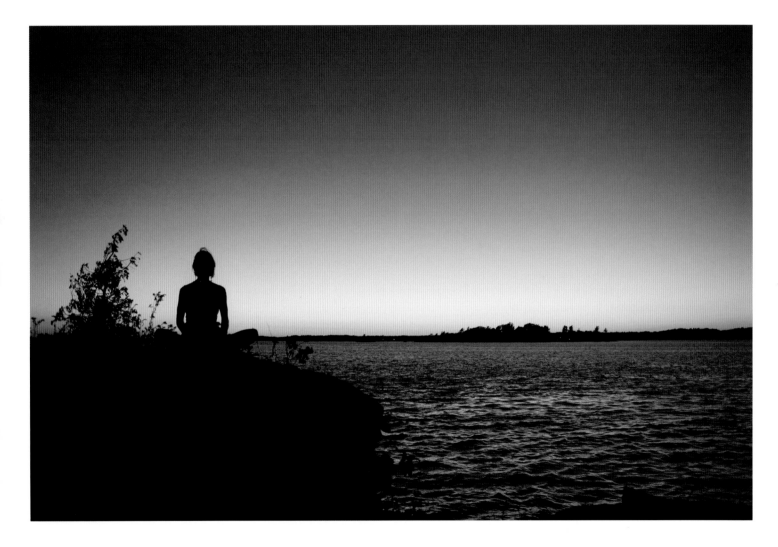

SAVOR

"We all eat, and it would be a sad waste of opportunity to eat badly."
ANNA THOMAS

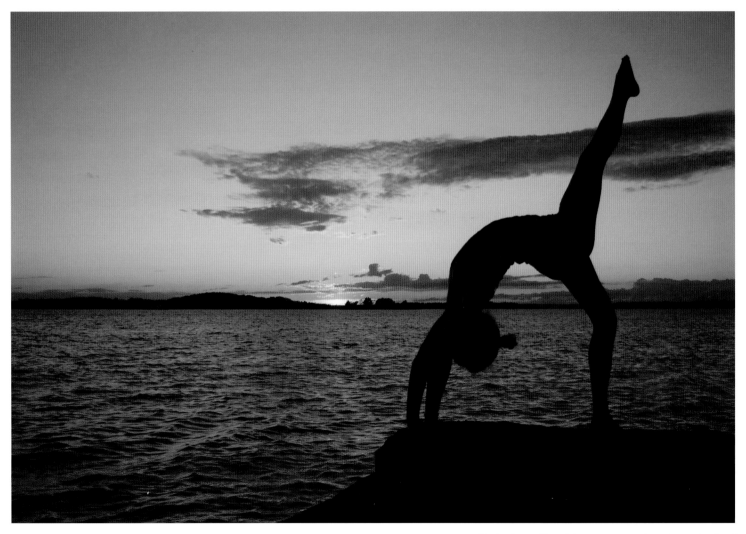

Eka Pada Urdhva Dhanurasana • One-Legged Wheel

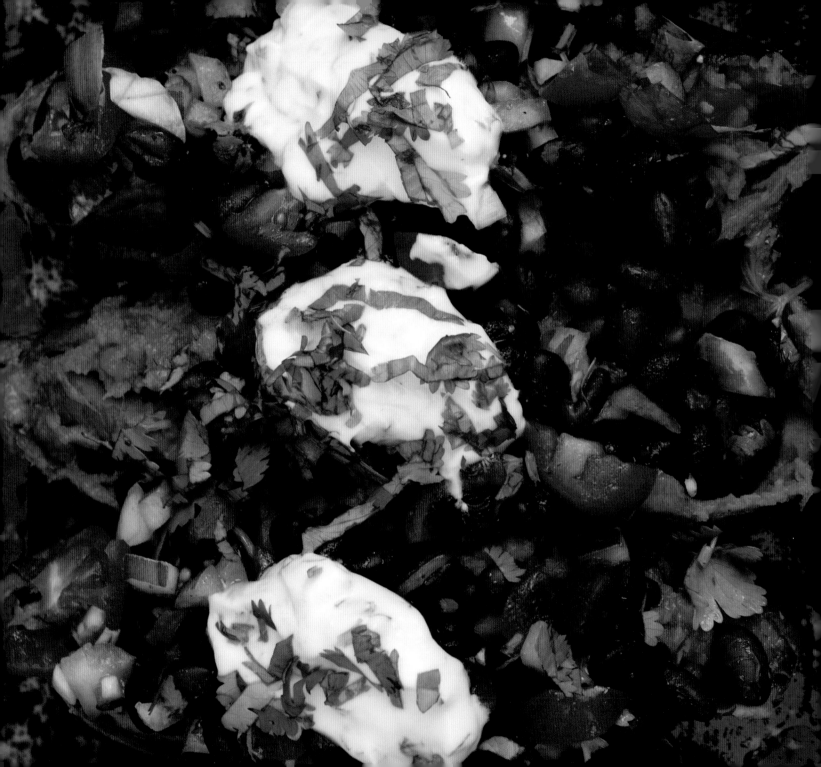

SWEET POTATO BURRITO BOATS *(v)*

Power up with these playful "boats," which are bursting with flavor and nutrition. This protein-rich Fresh Black Bean Salsa could be eaten on its own as well. Depending on how much sweet potato mash you want to put back into the "boats," leftovers could be used as a side dish for an entrée later in the week. Serves 4–8.

4 large sweet potatoes
½ tsp. olive oil
Himalayan salt coarsely ground (to taste)
Dash of cayenne
2T brown sugar

¼ cup cilantro (chopped)
1T lime juice
Himalayan salt coarsely ground (to taste)
Pepper coarsely ground (to taste)
1T olive oil

Fresh Black Bean Salsa
30 oz. black beans (rinsed and drained)
½ cup cherry tomatoes (diced)
¼ red onion (diced)
1 medium garlic clove (minced)
1 hot pepper (seeded, de-ribbed, and minced)

Yogurt Dressing (optional)
1 cup Greek yogurt
1T honey
1T olive oil
¼ cup cilantro

1. Preheat oven to 400°F.
2. Clean sweet potatoes, pierce each potato with fork a few times, and lightly coat with olive oil and salt.
3. Bake until sweet potatoes are cooked through or for about 1 hour.
4. Combine ingredients for *Fresh Black Bean Salsa*. Set aside.
5. Combine ingredients for *Yogurt Dressing*. Set aside in refrigerator.
6. When potatoes are cooked, carefully scoop out insides, hollowing out the shells and leaving about ⅛ inch of sweet potato lining along shells. With the sweet potato core, mash in a dash of cayenne and brown sugar. Equally distribute sweet potato mash among sweet potato shells.
7. Place *Fresh Black Bean Salsa* into sweet potato "boats."
8. Top with *Yogurt Dressing* (if desired). Serve.

NAVASANA
BOAT POSE

develops focus, improves digestion and coordination, strengthens core

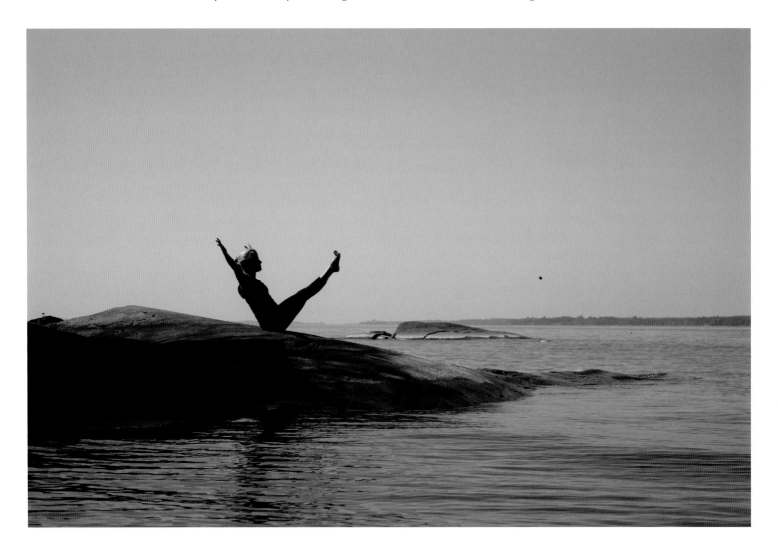

EFFORT

Through our practices we search for that fine line between effort and ease. Though postures often take great effort, our breath enables us to soften that effort, and the magic is discovered when we find that perfect space that allows us to just . . . be. Often in our practices, the true posture begins when we wish to leave it. Letting go of what we think we want, where we have been, or where we think we want to go, and discovering the beauty that is unveiled from being, is a lesson that transcends our yoga mats.

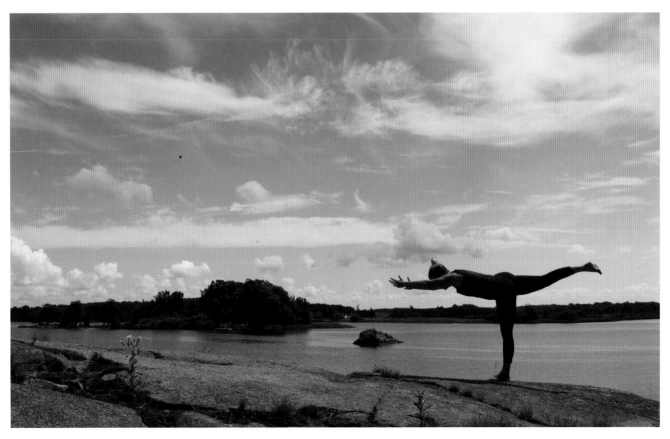

Virabhadrasana III • Warrior Pose Three

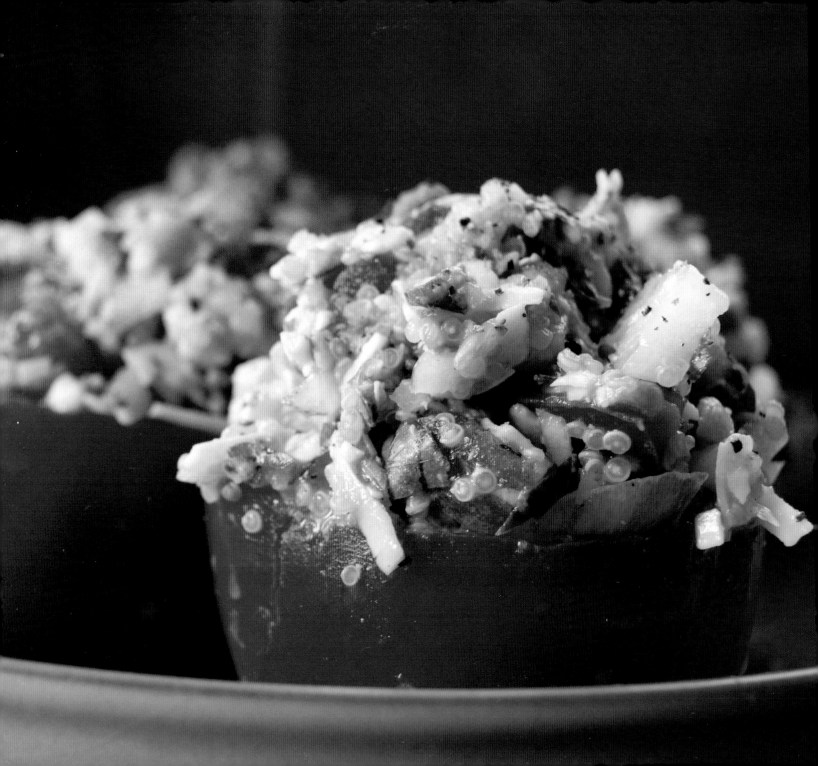

SATIATED (NOT-STUFFED) TOMATOES

Yoga teaches us to be aware and present in our postures. This awareness is also important when we are cooking and eating. Yogis eat healthy foods to nourish the body and mind. Awareness helps us to be mindful of what we put into our bodies and also the point when we become satiated—the point where we neither need more nor less. These Satiated (Not-Stuffed) Tomatoes contain ancient grains, nutritious parsley, and a mixture of cheeses. Serves 4.

4 large tomatoes
1 cup parsley (chopped)
4T lemon juice
½ red onion (chopped)
1 cup cooked quinoa (cooked per package instructions)
½ cup Gruyere (shredded)
½ cup sharp white cheddar (shredded)
Himalayan salt coarsely ground (to taste)
Pepper coarsely ground (to taste)
¼ cup Parmesan cheese (grated)
1T olive oil

1. Preheat oven to 375°F.
2. Remove stems from tomatoes.
3. Remove tops and core from tomatoes, leaving a stable but thin exterior tomato shell.
4. Place tomato insides in a medium mixing bowl and chop with knife and fork to create soup-like consistency. Combine with parsley, lemon juice, onion, quinoa, Gruyere, cheddar, salt, and pepper.
5. Scoop tomato mixture equally into four tomato shells. Top with equal amounts of grated Parmesan.
6. Drizzle 1 tablespoon of olive oil in a baking pan and place tomatoes in pan with stuffing side up.
7. Place pan in oven and bake for 40 minutes. Broil tomatoes for the last 30 seconds.
8. Remove from oven, plate, and serve immediately.

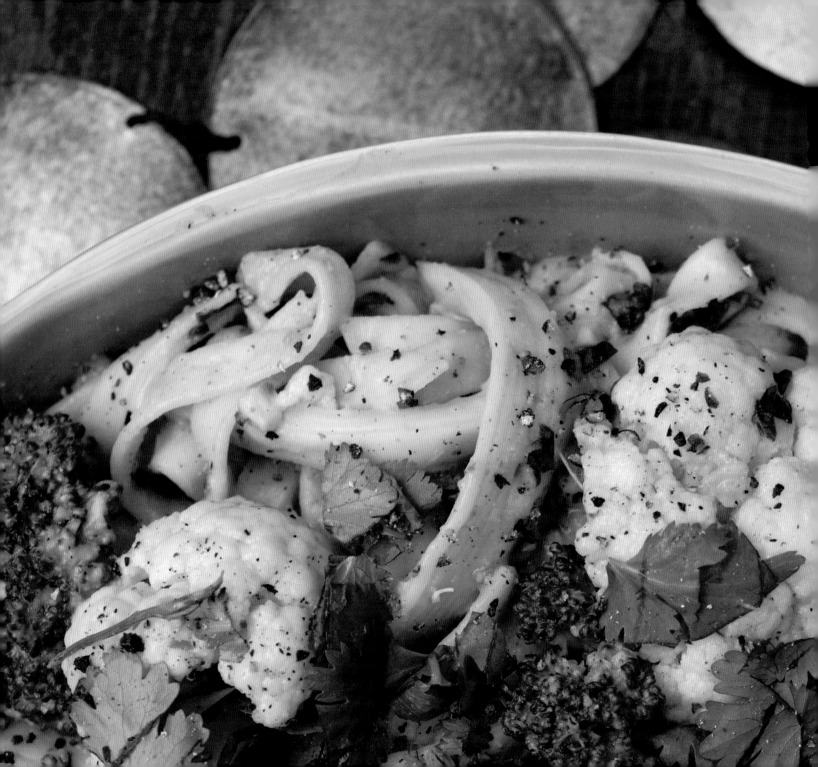

PASSIONATE PEANUT BUTTER NOODLES (v)

Surrender to the spiciness and sexiness of this dish. Though it may seem as though the list of ingredients for this dish is long, the truth is the peanut butter sauce for these noodles can be easily made with peanut butter, rice vinegar, and some spice. Be creative and feel free to explore variations and modifications! Our children and their friends love this dish (with a little less spice). Serves 8–10.

2T sesame seeds
1 cup peanut butter (crunchy or creamy)
1T sesame oil
2T tamari
4T rice vinegar
2T garlic chili paste (Asian style)
1T Asian-style hot sauce (if desired for extra heat)
2T brown sugar
3 medium garlic cloves (minced)
2T fresh ginger (minced)
1 medium jalapeño (seeded, de-ribbed, and minced)
2T lime juice
1 cup fresh cilantro (chopped)
2 cups fresh broccoli
2 cups fresh cauliflower
14 oz. rice noodles

1. Toast sesame seeds in skillet over medium-low heat until golden brown and fragrant.
2. Boil water in a medium saucepan over high heat.
3. Combine peanut butter, oil, tamari, rice vinegar, chili paste, hot sauce, sugar, garlic, ginger, jalapeño, and lime juice in medium bowl. Add ½ cup of fresh chopped cilantro to sauce. Set aside.
4. Boil broccoli and cauliflower for 4–5 minutes or until just tender. Carefully remove vegetables from water and allow to drain.
5. Cook pasta per package instructions or until al dente in same water. Drain well.
6. Combine peanut sauce, cooked noodles, and vegetables in large serving bowl.
7. Top with toasted sesame seeds and remaining ½ cup of cilantro. Serve.

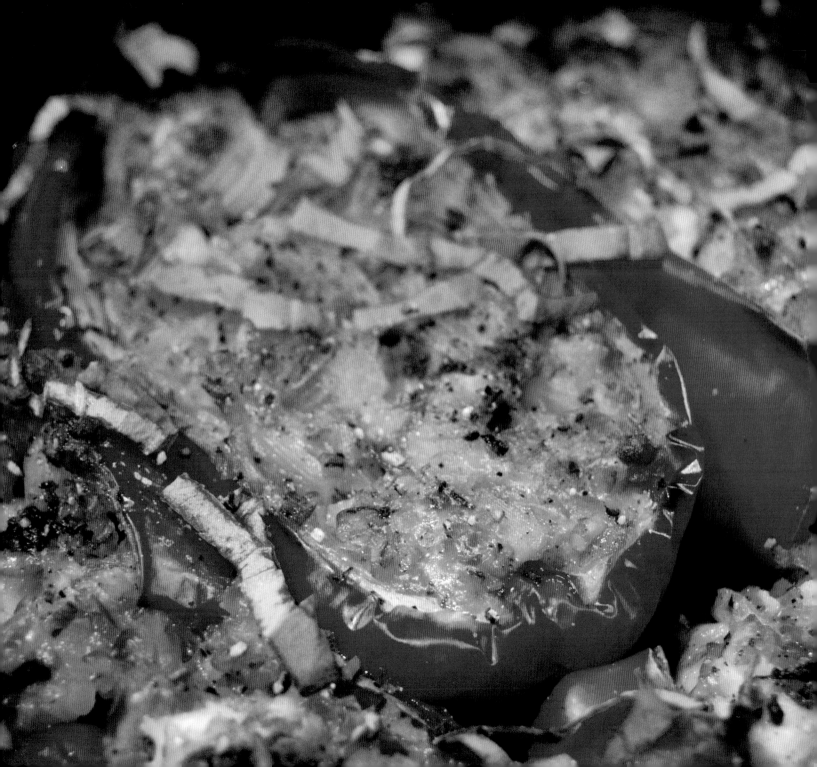

PLOUGH PEPPERS

Just as Plough Pose supports healthy immune functioning, so do our Plough Peppers. Red peppers are loaded with antioxidants and have potential anti-cancer benefits. Bulgar, sage, fennel, and spinach add to the healthfulness of these stuffed peppers. Serves 4.

4 bell peppers
1 cup cooked bulgar (cooked per package instructions)
2T olive oil
1 white onion (chopped)
5 medium garlic cloves (chopped)
2T fresh sage (chopped)
½ cup fennel (chopped)
Dash of cayenne pepper (to taste)
1 tsp. ground cumin
2 cups fresh spinach (chopped)
4 oz. canned or fresh green chili peppers (chopped)
Himalayan salt coarsely ground (to taste)
Pepper coarsely ground (to taste)
½ cup sharp white cheddar (shredded)
½ cup queso fresco (crumbled)
¼ cup goat cheese (crumbled)
½ cup thinly sliced basil leaves (garnish)

1. Preheat oven to 375°F.
2. Remove tops and cores from bell peppers.
3. Sauté onion and garlic with 1 tablespoon of olive oil in a medium skillet over low-medium heat for about 5 minutes or until softened. Add sage, fennel, cayenne, cumin, spinach, chili peppers, salt, and pepper and sauté for another 5 minutes.
4. Combine sautéed mixture with cooked bulgar and cheeses in a medium mixing bowl.
5. Spoon mixture equally into 4 pepper shells.
6. Pour remaining 1 tablespoon of olive oil in a baking pan and place stuffed peppers in pan with stuffing side up.
7. Place pan in oven and bake for about 1 hour or until peppers look slightly charred on edges. Broil peppers for the last minute.
8. Remove from oven, plate, garnish with basil and serve immediately.

HALASANA
PLOUGH POSE

supports immune functions, balances nervous system, brings symmetry to body

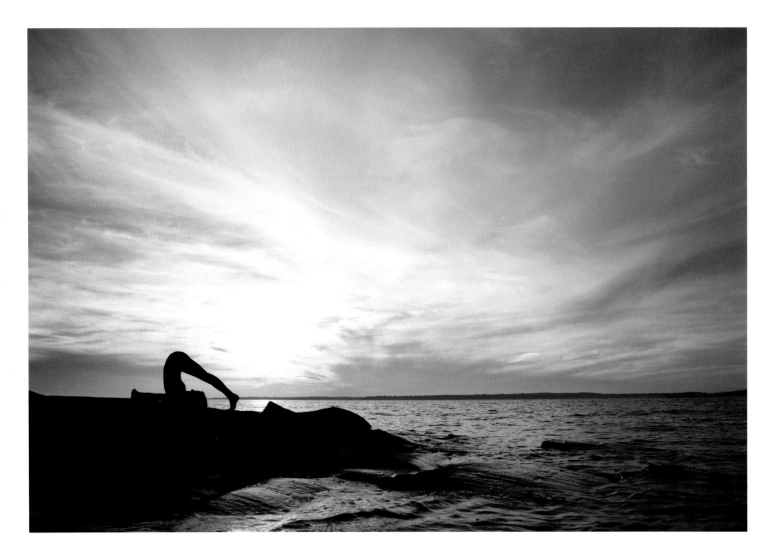

UTTHITA PARSVAKONASANA III
ADVANCED EXTENDED SIDE ANGLE POSE

strengthens and massages internal organs, detoxifies, opens the chest and lungs

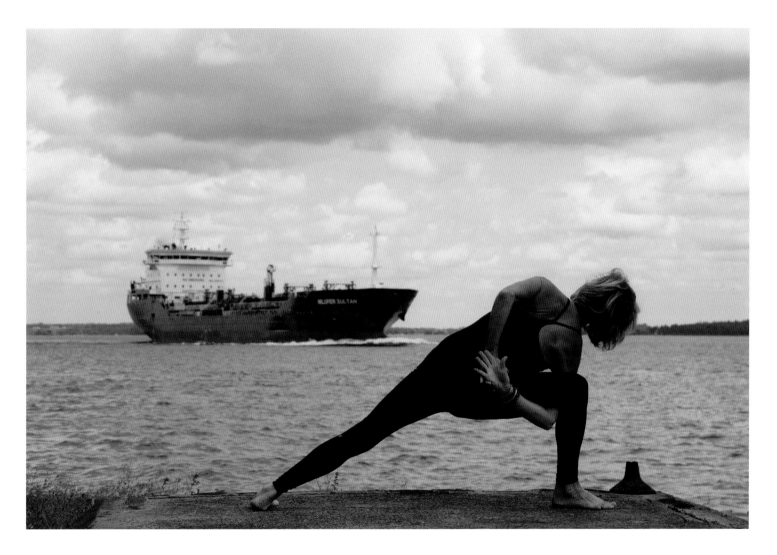

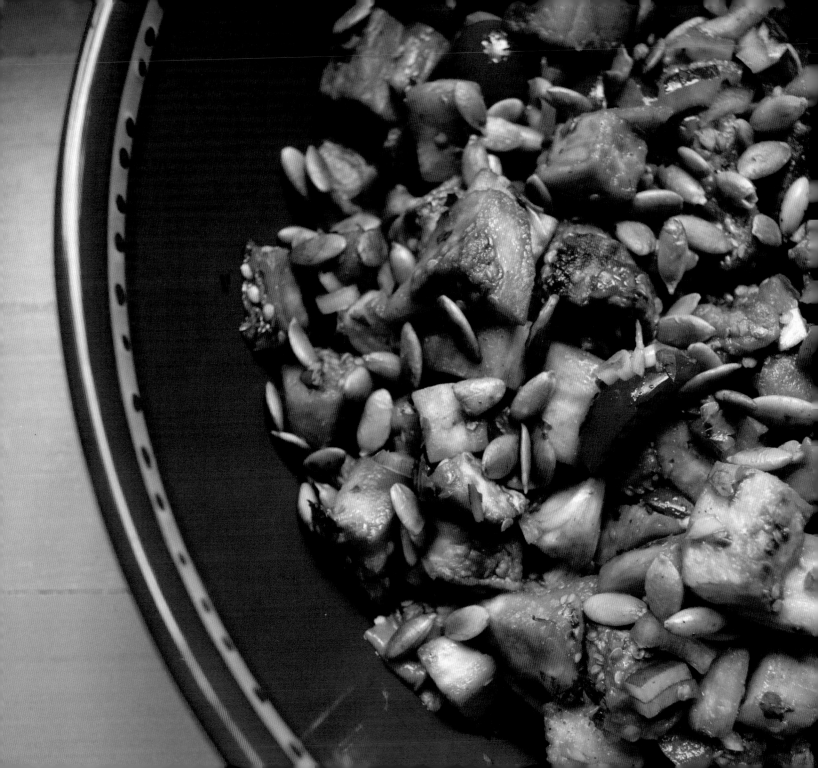

ELEVATED EGGPLANT (v)

The awareness we develop through our yoga practices encourages us to live more mindfully and spiritually elevated lives. There are not many better teachings than that! This isn't your traditional eggplant recipe (fried and drenched in mozzarella and tomato sauce). Though we love Eggplant Parmesan, we think we've taken our eggplant to the next level. We hope you find it elevated and very enjoyable!

3 large eggplants (peeled and cut into 1-inch squares)
¼ cup olive oil
1T pure maple syrup
6 medium garlic cloves (pressed)
½ tsp. ground toasted coriander
Dash of cayenne pepper
Himalayan salt coarsely ground (to taste)
Pepper coarsely ground (to taste)

1 cup cherry tomatoes (quartered or halved)

¼ cup red onion (chopped)
¼ cup scallions (chopped)
¼ cup flat parsley leaves (chopped)
¼ cup fresh cilantro (chopped)
1T orange juice
1T lime juice
1T agave nectar
2T tamari
2T olive oil

½ cup pepitas

1. Preheat oven to 400°F.
2. Sprinkle salt on cubed eggplant and let it sit for at least 10 minutes.
3. Prepare roasting marinade by combining olive oil, maple syrup, garlic, coriander, cayenne, salt, and pepper.
4. Rinse and pat eggplant dry and mix with marinade.
5. Place eggplant mixture on baking sheet in single layer. Roast for 30–40 minutes (tossing halfway through) or until eggplant is fork tender and golden brown. Remove from oven and allow to cool for at least 20 minutes.
6. Combine tomatoes, onion, scallions, parsley, and cilantro in a large bowl.
7. Make dressing by stirring together orange juice, lime juice, agave, tamari, and olive oil.
8. Toast pepitas in a skillet over low-medium heat until fragrant and golden brown. Remove from heat and set aside.
9. Combine cooled eggplant, tomato mixture, dressing, and toasted pepitas.
10. Serve slightly warm or at room temperature.

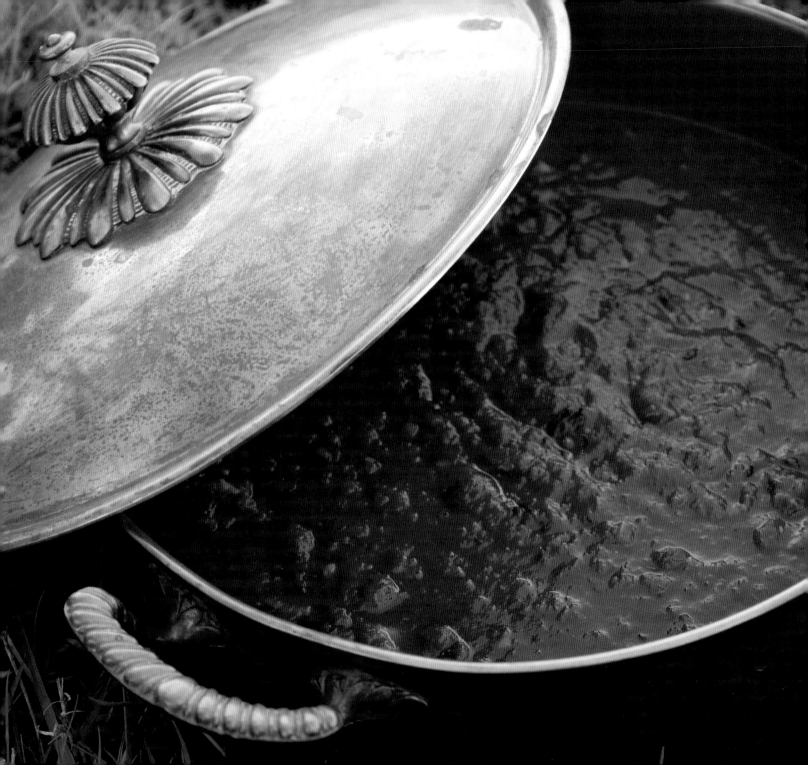

PLEASANT PEASANT TOMATO SAUCE (v)

The adage to "treat others the way you would like to be treated" is a great philosophy by which to live and one that sometimes slips our minds. Being pleasant and kind to others aligns seamlessly with the yoga philosophy of ahimsa (non-harming). Perfect with fresh pasta, this universal tomato sauce is a year-round favorite. Makes about 8 cups. Serves 8–10.

4T olive oil
2 medium yellow onions (chopped)
8 medium garlic cloves (chopped)
2 cups fresh basil (chopped)
2 bay leaves
½ tsp. hot red chili flakes
20–24 medium tomatoes (chopped) or 2 28 oz. cans diced tomatoes with juices
4T tomato paste
4T agave nectar
Himalayan salt coarsely ground (to taste)
Pepper coarsely ground (to taste)

Prepared fresh pasta (optional)

1. Heat olive oil in a Dutch oven or large saucepan over medium heat. Add onion and garlic and sauté for 5 to 10 minutes or until softened.
2. Add basil, bay leaves, chili flakes, tomatoes, tomato paste, agave, and salt and pepper to taste.
3. Simmer for about 30 minutes, stirring occasionally, until well combined.
4. Turn off heat. Remove bay leaves. Combine sauce slightly using an immersion blender.
5. Serve or allow to cool and store. This sauce may be stored in the refrigerator for up to 1 week or in the freezer for up to 3 months.

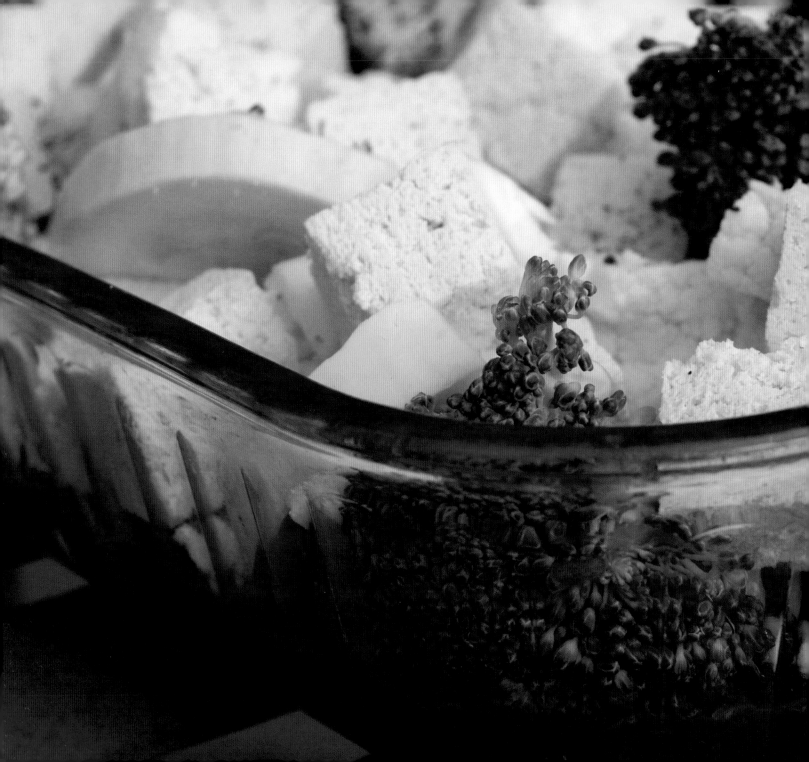

BANDHA BAKE *(v)*

Bandhas are "locks" that are meant to energize and tone the internal body. There are three main bandhas—Mula Bandha (root), Uddiyana Banda (core), and Jhalandara Bandha (chin)—and also "the great lock" (Maha Bandha), which is when we activate all three main bandhas at the same time. Our Bandha Bake is packed with fresh vegetables and tofu. This protein-rich dish was designed to fuel the body and mind. If you make the Ginger Glow dressing ahead of time, this recipe has limited prep time. Variation: Serve Bandha Bake over sautéed kale, onions, and garlic instead of rice. Serves 8.

1½ cups *Ginger Glow* dressing (see recipe on page 158)

1 12 oz. package super firm tofu (frozen then completely thawed)
1 large yellow onion (chopped)
3 medium garlic cloves (chopped)
2 heads fresh broccoli (cut from stalk and lightly chopped)
1 head cauliflower (cut from stalk and lightly chopped)
1 yellow squash (sliced)
Himalayan salt coarsely ground (to taste)
Pepper coarsely ground (to taste)

2 cups brown rice
2 cups coconut milk
2 cups water
2T red curry paste

½ cup cilantro (chopped)

1. Preheat oven to 350°F.
2. Prepare *Ginger Glow* dressing recipe. Set aside.
3. Squeeze out tofu liquid and cut tofu into ½-inch cubes.
4. Combine tofu with onion, garlic, broccoli, cauliflower, squash, and *Ginger Glow* dressing.
5. Place mixture in a large baking pan and place in oven for about 1 hour, stirring half way through cooking time.
6. With about 30–45 minutes left in cooking tofu vegetable bake, start making rice. Bring coconut milk, water, and curry to a boil. Add brown rice. Bring to a boil and then reduce heat. Cover and simmer for about 30–45 minutes or until rice is cooked and liquid is absorbed.
7. Place ½ cup or 1 full cup of rice on each plate. Top with 1 cup of the tofu vegetable bake. Top with equal amounts of cilantro. Serve immediately.

SETU BANDHASANA
BRIDGE POSE

rejuvenating, exhilarating, stimulates thyroid glands

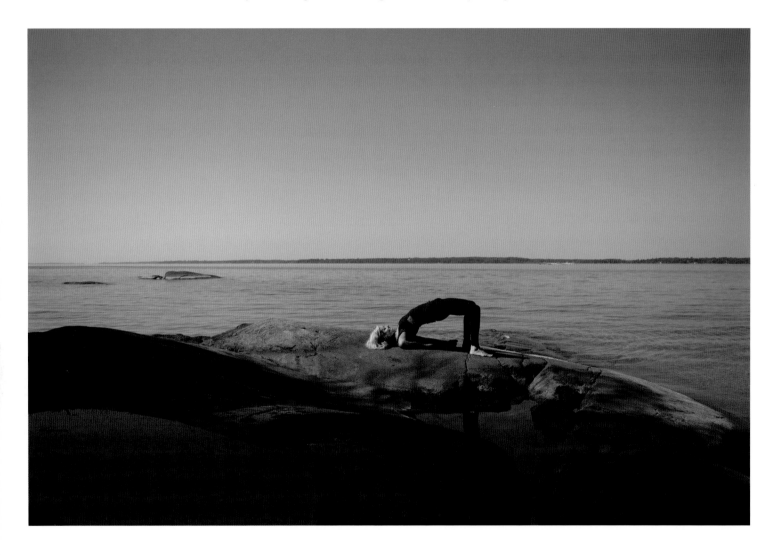

CONTENTMENT (SANTOSA)

"To live content with small means; to seek elegance rather than luxury, and refinement rather than fashion, to be worthy, not respectable, and wealthy, not rich; to study hard, think quietly, talk gently, act frankly, to listen to stars and birds, to babes and sages, with open heart, to bear all cheerfully, to all bravely await occasions, hurry never. In a word, to let the spiritual unbidden and unconscious grow up through the common. This is to be my symphony."
WILLIAM HENRY CHANNING

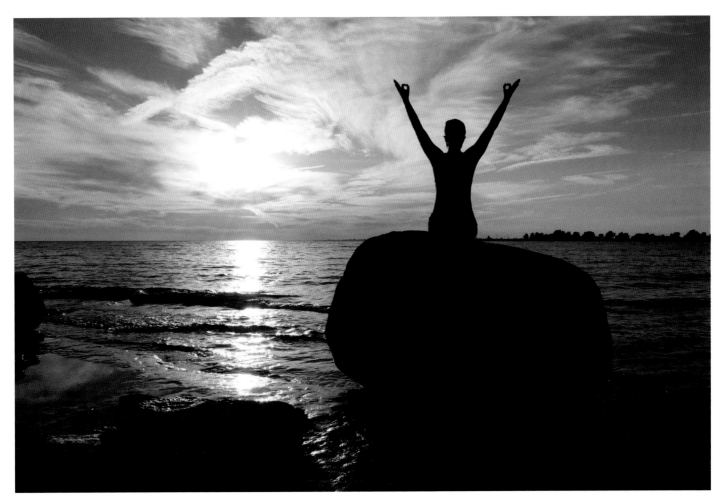

Gyan or Chin Mudra • Hand Gesture Representing Unified Consciousness

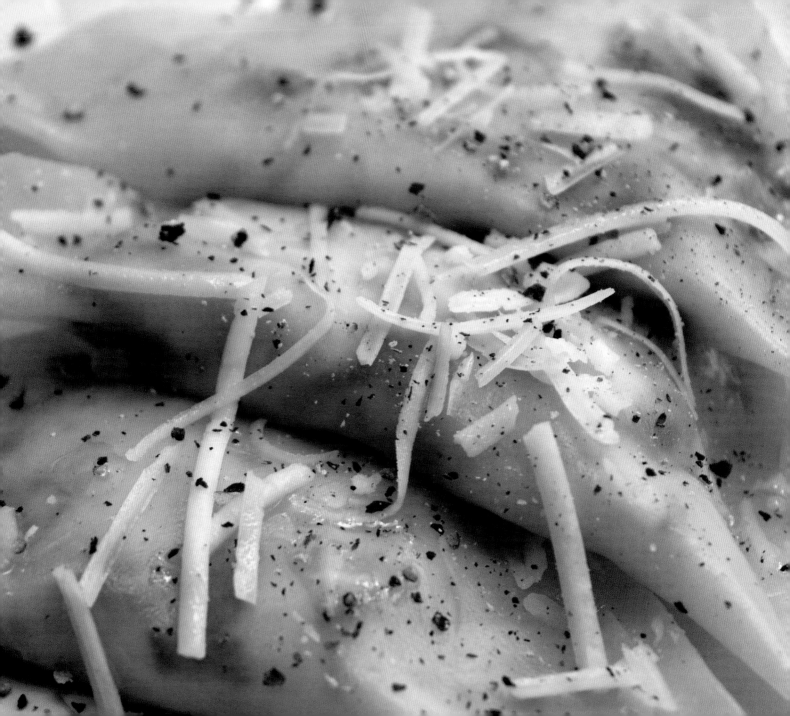

WEALTHY WONTON PURSES

"Health is the greatest gift, contentment the greatest wealth, faithfulness the best relationship."
SIDDHARTHA GAUTAMA

To a true yogi, material possessions may be superfluous, unwanted. Wealth is found in terms of seemingly intangible riches, such as joy, love, community, compassion, and ultimately, fulfillment. We have created two variations of our Wealthy Wonton Purses—one contains cheese and the other is vegan. Each recipe variation makes 18–20 purses and serves 4.

CHEESE LOVERS
1T olive oil
2 medium garlic cloves (pressed)
½ medium white onion (minced)
2 cups fresh spinach (chopped)
2T fresh tarragon (chopped)
1T fresh basil (chopped)
Dash of nutmeg
½ cup ricotta cheese
½ cup grated Romano cheese

Dash of cayenne pepper
Himalayan salt coarsely ground (to taste)
18–20 wonton wraps

Topping
Himalayan salt coarsely ground (to taste)
Pepper coarsely ground (to taste)
2T olive oil
Grated Parmesan cheese (to taste)

1. In a large skillet over medium heat, sauté garlic and onion until softened or for about 5 minutes.
2. Add spinach, tarragon, and basil. Cook for another 5 minutes or until spinach is wilted.
3. Take mixture off of heat and add nutmeg, ricotta, Romano, cayenne, and salt to taste.
4. Place 1 small tablespoon of the mixture onto the center of each wrapper. Wet all four edges of the wraps with water using your index finger. Fold the filled wraps into triangles. Press the edges of the wraps together with the prongs of a fork.
5. Carefully place the *Wealthy Wonton Purses* in a large saucepan of boiling water. Boil for about 1 minute. With a slotted spoon, gently remove the wontons from the water.
6. Place 4 to 5 cooked wontons on each plate. Top with salt and pepper to taste, drips of olive oil, and Parmesan cheese. Serve immediately.

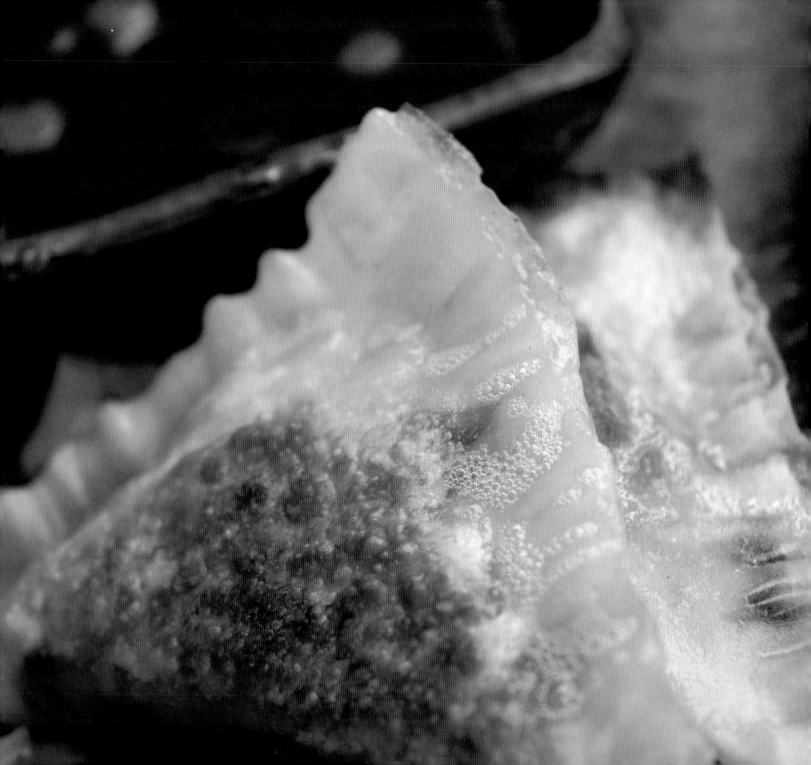

WEALTHY WONTON PURSES (continued)

ASIAN STYLE *(v)*

Sauce

2T tamari
2T rice vinegar
1T sesame oil
1T Hoisin sauce
1T agave nectar
1T scallions (chopped)

1T olive oil
2 medium garlic cloves (minced)

½ medium red onion (minced)
2T fresh ginger (minced)
½ cup dried Asian mushrooms (reconstituted, drained, and minced)
½ cup bok choy (minced)
½ cup fresh cilantro (chopped)
½ tsp. tamari
Ground coriander (to taste)
Ground white pepper (to taste)
18–20 wonton wraps
2T sesame oil

1. Prepare sauce by combining all ingredients. Divide into four small dipping bowls. Set aside.
2. In a large skillet over medium heat, sauté garlic, onion, and ginger in olive oil until softened or for about 5 minutes.
3. Add mushrooms and bok choy and sauté for an additional 5 minutes.
4. Add cilantro, tamari, coriander, and white pepper. Combine and remove mixture from heat.
5. Place 1 small tablespoon of the mixture onto the center of each wrapper. Wet all four edges of the wraps with water using your index finger. Fold the filled wraps into triangles. Press the edges of the wraps together with the prongs of a fork.
6. Place sesame oil in a large skillet over medium heat. Pan sear *Asian Style Wealthy Wonton Purses* for 2 to 3 minutes on each side or until slightly golden brown.
7. Add 2 tablespoons of water to pan and place a lid over the pan to allow *Purses* to steam.
8. Arrange 4 to 5 wontons on each plate. Serve immediately with dipping sauce.

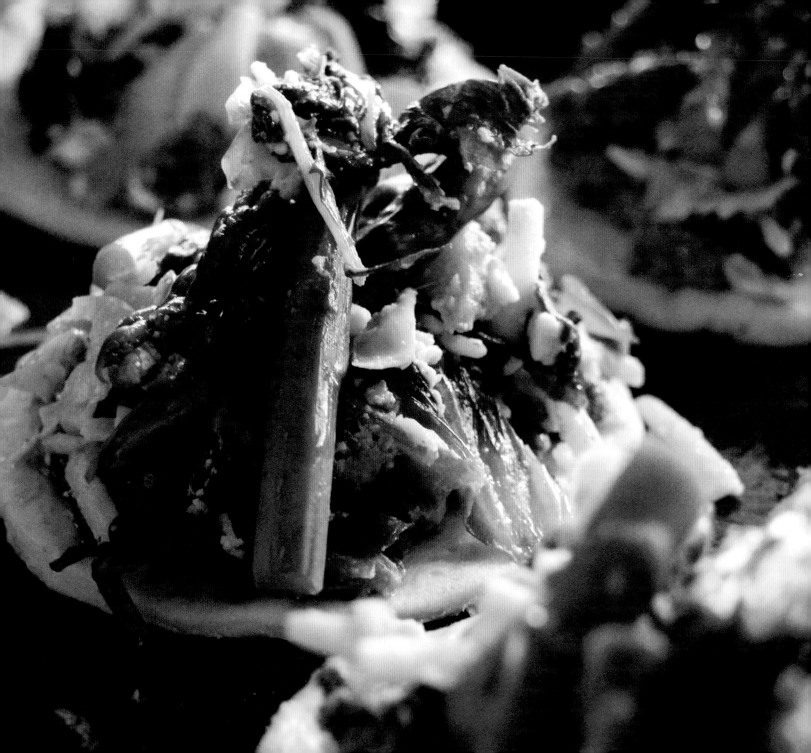

HIDDEN TREASURE

Whether you embark on your yoga journey to lose weight, gain flexibility, for spiritual guidance, or for any other reason, you are developing a practice of mindful being that will help to bring balance, joy, and love into your life. Twenty-five years ago, when Liz started practicing yoga, you could say that yoga was a bit of a "hidden treasure" in the United States. Though quickly becoming more and more popular, yoga is still a true treasure, and those who embrace the philosophies of yoga are very fortunate.

Underneath an envelope of flaky puff pastry awaits a treasure of beautiful vegetables and cheeses for your delight! Serves 4.

4 oz. pesto (see *Prana Pesto* recipe on page 46)
1 lb. asparagus (cut to use 3-inch tips only)
2T olive oil
2 medium garlic cloves (minced)
1 large shallot (minced)
2 cups packed fresh spinach (chopped)
1T tarragon (chopped)
1T thyme (chopped)
Dash of hot pepper flakes
Himalayan salt coarsely ground (to taste)

Pepper coarsely ground (to taste)
½ cup canned artichoke hearts (drained and chopped)
½ cup sundried tomatoes (chopped)
½ cup feta cheese (crumbled)
½ cup Gruyere (shredded)
1 package puff pastry (partially thawed)
16 oz. marinara sauce (see *Pleasant Peasant Tomato Sauce* recipe on page 225)

1. Preheat oven to 400°F.
2. In a large pot of boiling water, cook the asparagus for 1 to 2 minutes or until just tender. Drain and rinse with cold water. Set aside.
3. In a medium skillet over medium heat, sauté garlic and shallot in olive oil for about 3 minutes. Add spinach, tarragon, thyme, hot pepper flakes, and salt and pepper to taste. Sauté for an additional 5 minutes. Remove from heat.
4. Stir mixture in a large mixing bowl, adding artichokes, tomatoes, and cheeses.
5. Prepare puff pastry. Using a rolling pin, create 4 ⅛-inch-thick and 5 inches in diameter, rounds of pastry. Then, create 4 ⅛-inch-thick and 7 inches in diameter, rounds of pastry.
6. On a lightly greased baking sheet arrange the 4 5-inch rounds of pastry (leaving 1 inch between rounds). Spread pesto on pastry leaving a ¼-inch border. Top with ⅛ of the spinach mixture. Add ¼ of the asparagus on top in a single layer. Top with another ⅛ of the spinach mixture. Top each round with a 7-inch round of pastry.
7. Press edges of pastry together using the back of a fork. Pierce tops of *Treasures* with fork.
8. Bake for about 30 minutes or until golden brown.
9. Remove immediately and serve one *Hidden Treasure* surrounded by marinara sauce to each diner. Enjoy.

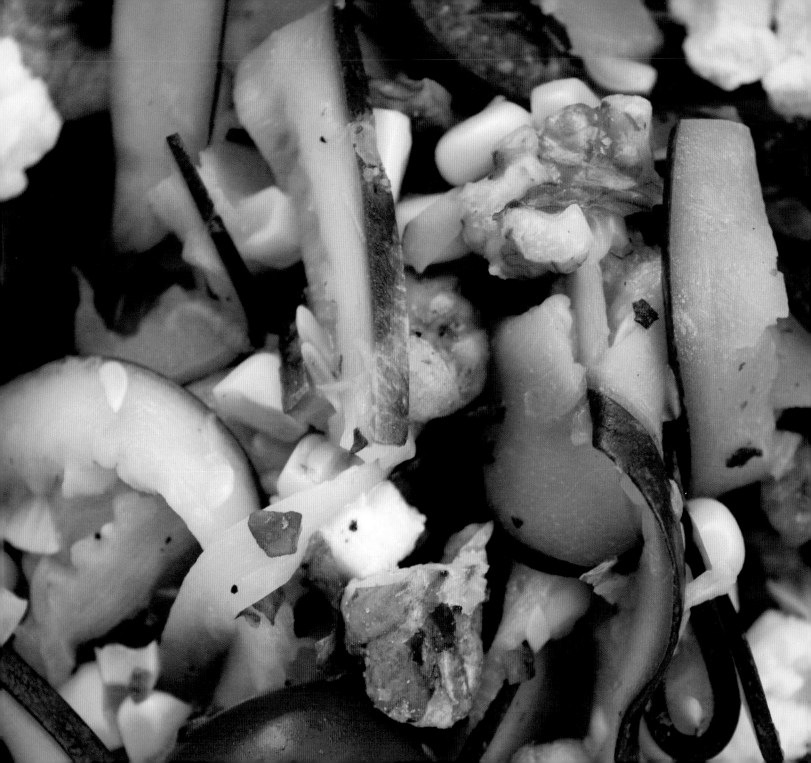

LOVEEE ZUCCHINI LINGUINI *(v)*

"The most precious gift we can offer anyone is our attention. When mindfulness embraces those we love, they will bloom like flowers." THICH NHAT HANH

You won't even begin to miss traditional pasta. . . Our Loveee Zucchini Linguini, named after our fellow yogi and family member, is a great dinner option for families. Kids seem to love the playful zucchini noodles. This is a great summer dish. It is colorful, light, and totally delicious. Serves 4.

½ cup walnuts
2T olive oil
2 medium garlic cloves (minced)
½ shallot (minced)
4 cups julienned zucchini
1T oregano (chopped)
1T tarragon (chopped)
1 cup fresh corn kernels
½ cup cherry tomatoes
½ cup crumbled goat cheese (optional)
Himalayan salt coarsely ground (to taste)
Pepper coarsely ground (to taste)

1. Toast nuts in a medium skillet over low-medium heat, adding salt to taste throughout the process, until golden brown and fragrant. Remove from heat and set aside.
2. In a medium skillet over medium heat, sauté garlic and shallot in olive oil for about 3 minutes. Add zucchini, oregano, and tarragon and sauté for an additional 5–10 minutes or until slightly tender.
3. Turn off heat and stir in corn, tomatoes, goat cheese, toasted nuts, and salt and pepper to taste.
4. Divide into 4 portions on plates and serve immediately.

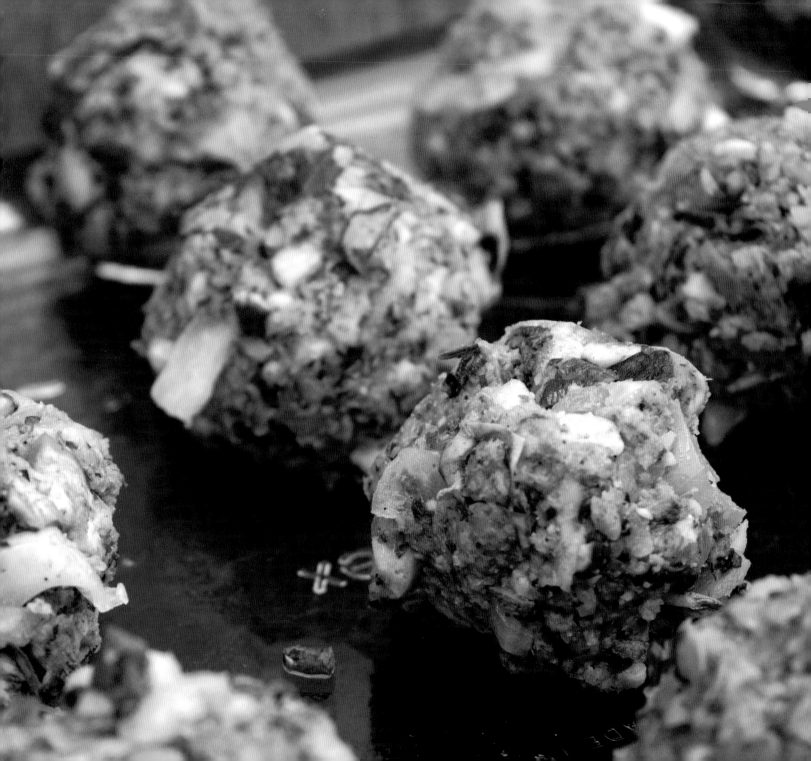

"BALL"ASANAS (v)

Balasana, which is also called Child's Pose or Wisdom Pose, is a restorative posture that allows the body to soften and surrender. Our "Ball"asanas are comforting, feel-good food. They are super hearty and satiating vegan meatballs. Enjoy them when you want to relax and spend time with friends and family. Makes about 20 balls. Serves 4–5.

8 oz. dried porcini mushrooms
½ medium yellow onion (chopped)
½ medium orange bell pepper (core removed, seeded, de-ribbed, and chopped)
4 medium garlic cloves (chopped)
Dash of cayenne pepper
1 tsp. fresh oregano (chopped)
2T fresh basil (chopped)
1 tsp. fresh thyme (chopped)
½ tsp. fresh sage (chopped)
1 cup seasoned breadcrumbs
¼ cup raw pecans (chopped)

3T pesto (see *Prana Pesto* recipe on page 46)
2T tomato paste
Himalayan salt coarsely ground (to taste)
Pepper coarsely ground (to taste)
1T olive oil

Optional Accompaniments
Freshly grated Parmesan cheese
Tomato sauce (see *Pleasant Peasant Tomato Sauce* recipe on page 222)
Fresh basil leaves
Cooked pasta

1. Preheat oven to 400°F.
2. Reconstitute porcini mushrooms per package instructions. Drain mushrooms and reserve liquid. Chop mushrooms.
3. Combine chopped porcini mushrooms with remaining ingredients (excluding olive oil and garnishes) in a large mixing bowl.
4. Take half the mixture and place it in a food processor. Pulse a few times and then recombine with original mixture.
5. Evenly distribute olive oil in bottom of a large baking dish.
6. Take about 2 tablespoons of ball mixture and shape into a round ball. Place in baking dish. Continue this process until mixture is gone.
7. Bake balls in the oven, uncovered, for about 30 to 45 minutes. The "Ball"asanas should look brown and crisp on the outside, but still be juicy on the inside.
8. Serve with desired accompaniments.

BALASANA
CHILD'S POSE

physical, mental, and emotional relief,
calming, aids in steady breathing

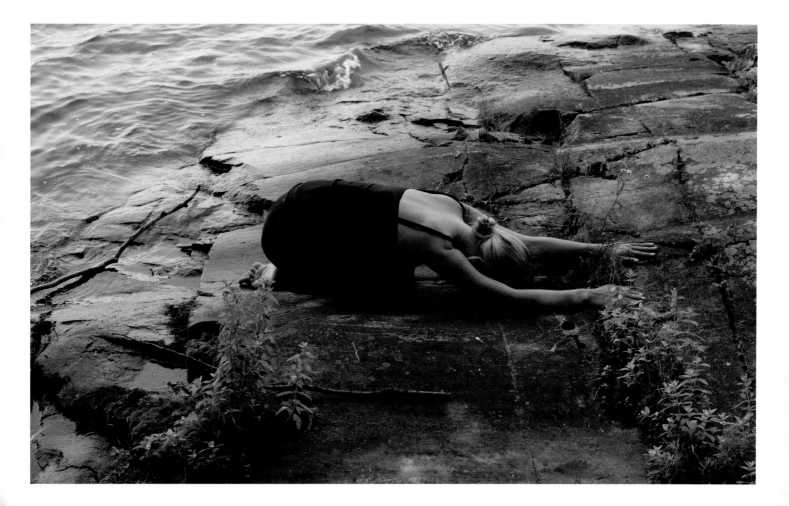

TRANSITION

Often, transitions are viewed as a means of getting from one thing to the next and may therefore be met with hurry, angst, anxiety, fear, or mindlessness. How often have we driven in a car and not remembered the journey, hurried through a yoga sequence just to get to another posture, or quickly "grabbed" a bite to eat before running out the door? This kind of mindless movement creates an illusion of separation from one movement or activity to the next. It blinds us to the beauty of the transition. Transitions are moments to be celebrated. They are *postures,* and if given attention, they will reveal more to us than what came before and whatever is coming next.

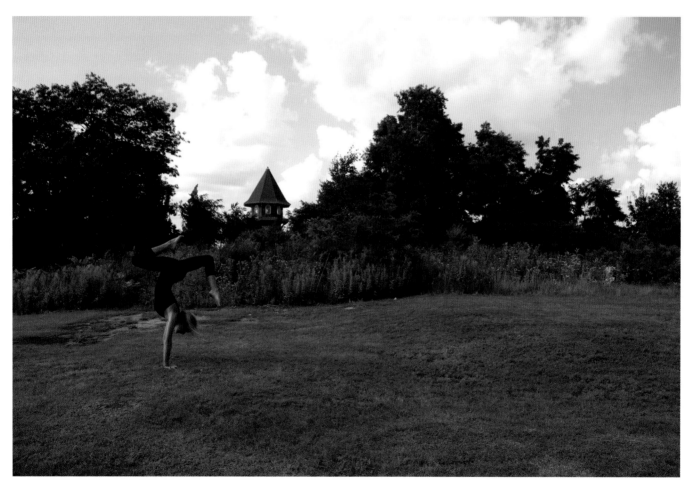

Adho Mukha Vrksasana • Handstand

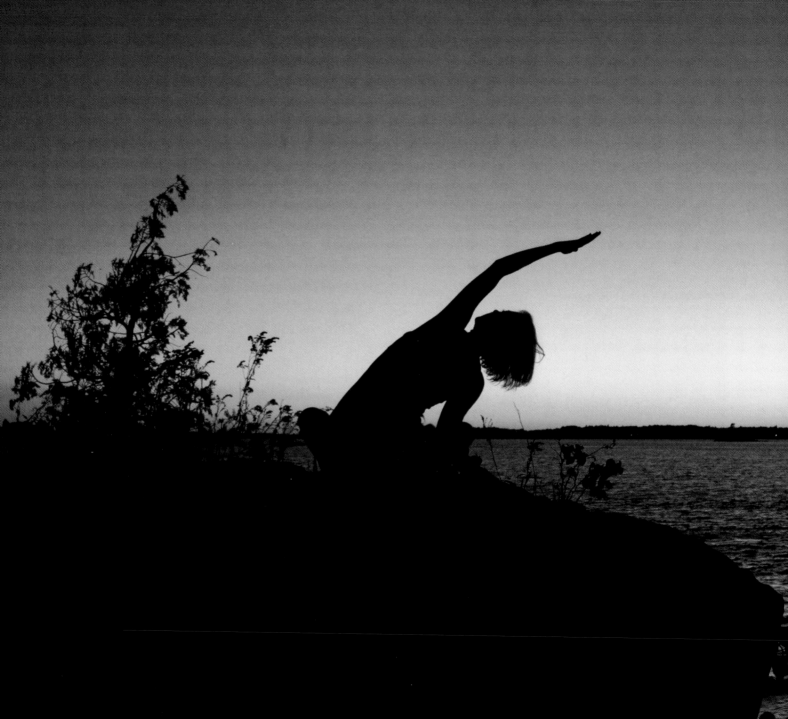

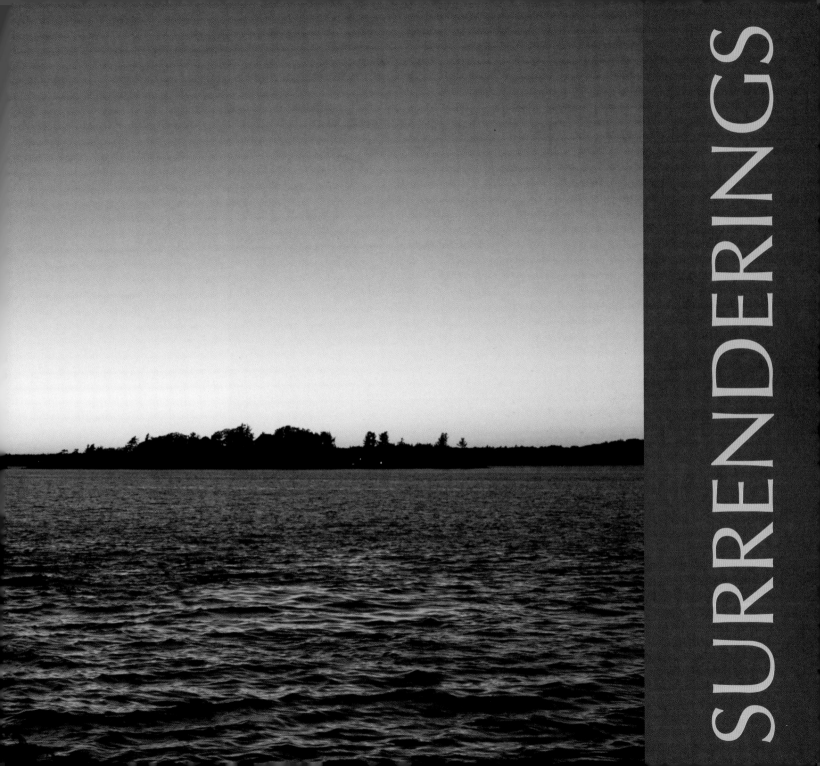

SURRENDERINGS

SURRENDER

"Empty the cup."
ZEN MASTER NAN-IN

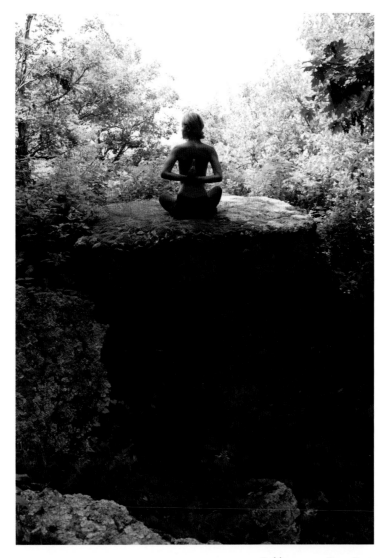

Sukhasana • Easy Pose

WASHING THE DISHES TO WASH THE DISHES

"At first glance that might seem a little silly: Why put so much stress on a simple thing? But that's precisely the point. The fact that I am standing there washing the bowls is a wondrous reality. I'm being completely myself, following my breath, conscious of my presence, and conscious of my thoughts and actions. There's no way I can be tossed around mindlessly like a bottle slapped here and there on the waves."

THICH NHAT HANH

Parivrtta Trikonasana • Revolved Triangle Pose

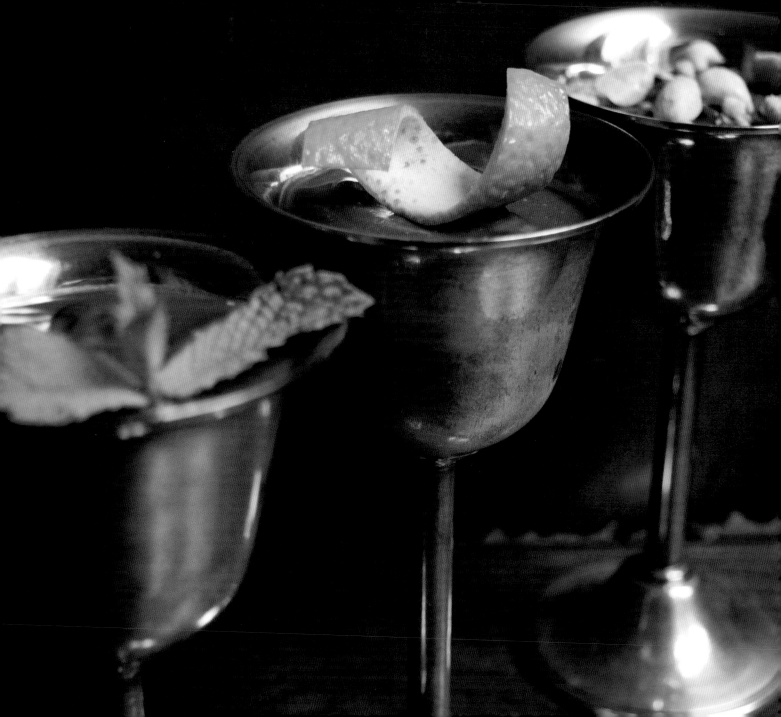

MOUSSE MOUNTAINS *(v)*

All of our desserts are no-bake, making them very simple to make. For when you feel like you need a little bit of extra surrender and balance, indulge in these chocolate-lovers' tofu-based chocolate mousses. For vegan variations, choose vegan chocolate chips. These desserts are easy and divine. Each recipe serves 4–8.

CITRUS
1 lb. silken tofu (room temperature)
10 oz. (1 bag) premium dark or semi-sweet chocolate chips
1 tsp. pure vanilla (optional)
5–7 drops pure food grade orange essential oil
Himalayan salt coarsely ground (to taste)
Garnish with orange peel

GRASSHOPPER
1 lb. silken tofu (room temperature)
10 oz. (1 bag) premium dark or semi-sweet chocolate chips
1 tsp. pure vanilla (optional)
4 drops pure food grade peppermint essential oil
¼ tsp. Himalayan salt (coarsely ground) or to taste
Garnish with fresh mint leaves

SINFULLY SUBLIME
1 lb. silken tofu (room temperature)
10 oz. (1 bag) milk chocolate chips
1 cup smooth peanut butter
Garnish with ¼ cup unsalted peanuts (roasted with sea salt to taste and chopped)

1. Puree tofu in blender or mixer.
2. Melt chocolate chips over double boiler, stirring constantly.
3. Add remaining ingredients of *Mousse Mountain* variety of choice.
4. Pour chocolate mixture over pureed tofu in blender or mixer and blend with tofu until smooth, fully combined, and lightened slightly in color.
5. Transfer mousse into individual serving dishes (possibly martini glasses) and immediately cool in refrigerator for at least 2 hours. Garnish as appropriate before serving. Serve cold.

TADASANA
MOUNTAIN POSE

foundational, improves posture, focuses awareness, promotes harmony

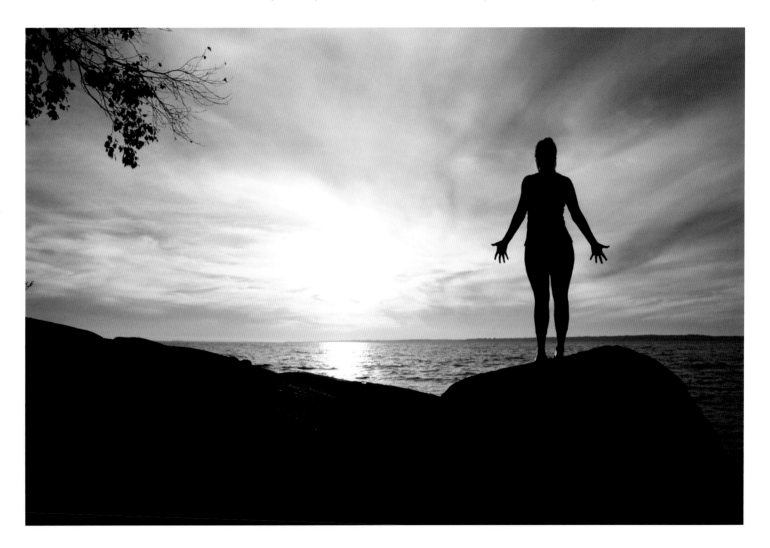

PARSVA BHUJA DANDASANA
GRASSHOPPER

nourishes spine, strengthens core

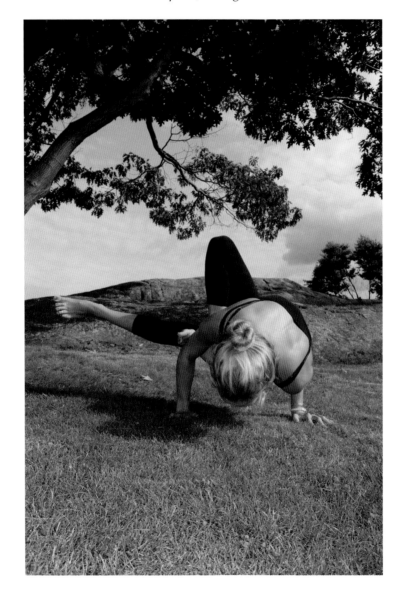

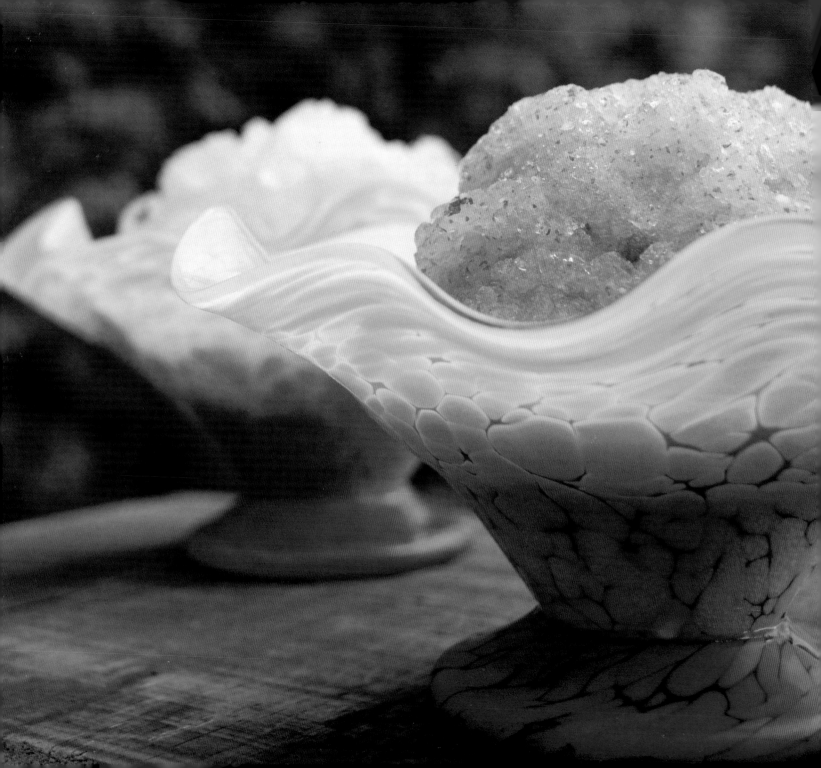

DELIGHTFULLY SILLY SNOW CONES *(v)(r)*

As the name of these desserts implies, they are light and joyful. How you eat your Delightfully Silly Snow Cones is up to you! Feeling refined? Serve the ice in 2 hollowed, frozen lemon halves. Feeling playful? Serve them in paper snow cone wrappers. Feeling like our friend Nancy? Simply serve them with a spoon. Served any way, these are totally refreshing, enjoyable, and healthy treats. They also make great palate cleansers. Serves 4.

LIGHT-FILLED LEMON

1T fresh ginger
1T fresh basil
5T lemon juice
3T agave nectar
3 cups crushed ice

1. In a food processor, mince ginger and basil.
2. Add lemon juice and agave nectar. Mix with ingredients.
3. Add crushed ice. Combine until mixture is slushy and no large ice chunks remain.
4. Serve as desired.

OVER-THE-MOON ORANGE

1T fresh ginger
1T fresh cilantro
4T lime juice
3T honey or agave nectar
3T fresh orange juice
3 cups crushed ice

1. In a food processor, mince ginger and cilantro.
2. Add lime juice, honey, and orange juice. Mix with ingredients.
3. Add crushed ice. Combine until mixture is slushy and no large ice chunks remain.
4. Serve as desired.

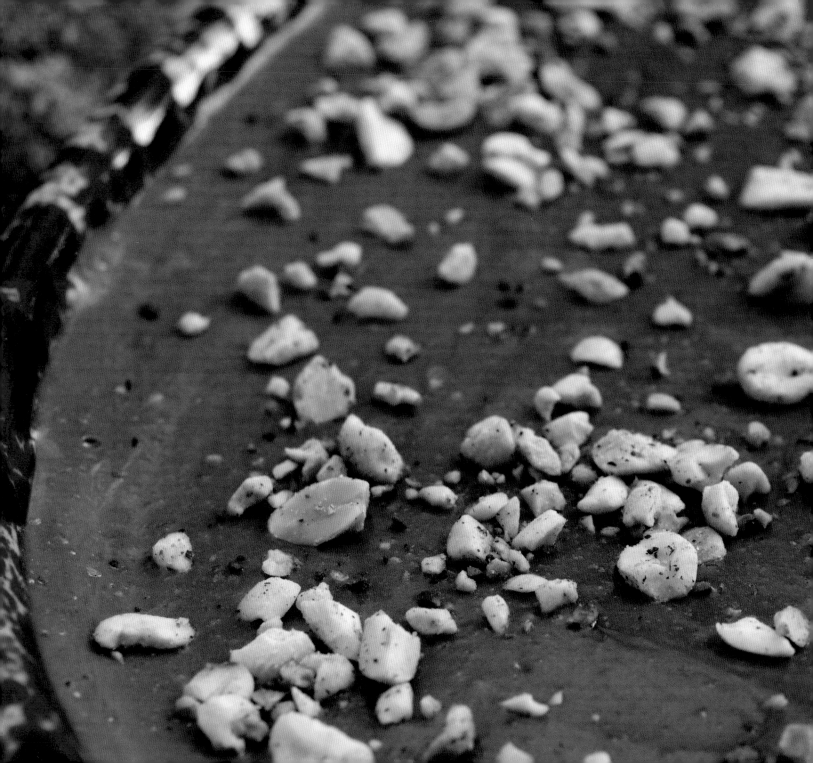

SINFULLY SUBLIME PIE

Wow! This recipe is a winner! We shared this prepared pie with a group of non-vegan family members, and it was totally revered. The toasted nut piecrust nourishes the soul. Sinfully Sublime Pie is a wonderfully light, yet decadent, treat, and we think sharing this pie with your neighbors, kids, families, and friends is a true token of love. Serves 12–16.

No-Bake Pie Crust
1 cup pecans (toasted and chopped)
1 cup raw almonds (toasted and chopped)
½ cup light brown sugar (packed)
3T olive oil
Himalayan salt coarsely ground, to taste (for toasted pecans)

Sinfully Sublime Mousse Mountain (see recipe on page 244)

1. Toast nuts in a medium skillet over low-medium heat, adding salt to taste throughout the process, until golden brown and fragrant. Remove from heat and set aside.
2. Process toasted nuts in food processor with brown sugar and olive oil.
3. Press mixture into the bottom of a pie dish or 8 x 8 inch glass baking dish. Cool in the refrigerator.
4. Prepare *Sinfully Sublime Mousse Mountain* recipe. Pour mousse directly on top of piecrust and refrigerate for at least two hours. Before serving, top with toasted peanuts according to *Sinfully Sublime Mousse Mountain* recipe.

PASSION

"If it's wild to your own heart, protect it. Preserve it. Love it. And fight for it, and dedicate yourself to it, whether it's a mountain range, your wife, your husband, or even (god forbid) your job. It doesn't matter if it's wild to anyone else: if it's what makes your heart sing, if it's what makes your days soar like a hawk in the summertime, then focus on it. Because for sure, it's wild, and if it's wild, it'll mean you're still free. No matter where you are."
RICK BASS (*WILD TO THE HEART*)

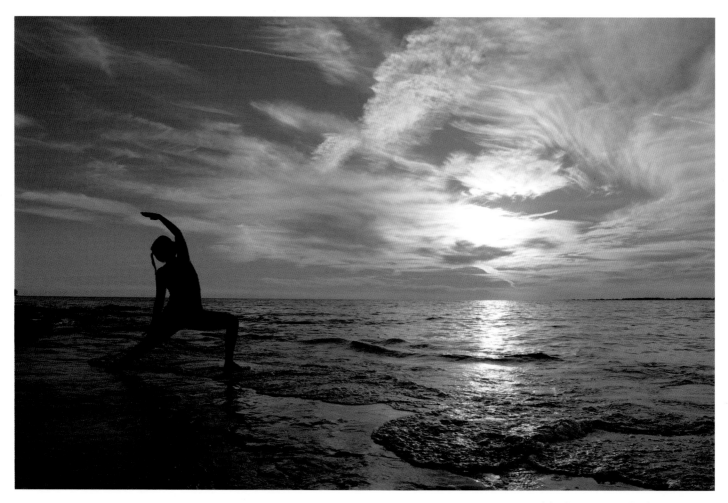

Viparita Virabhadrasana • Exalted Warrior Pose

TRIKONASANA
TRIANGLE POSE

*calming as well as energizing,
promotes flexibility of hips*

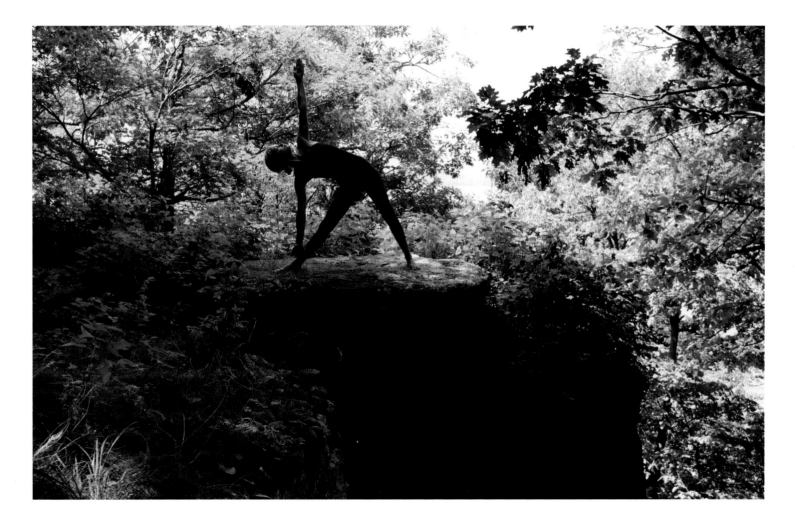

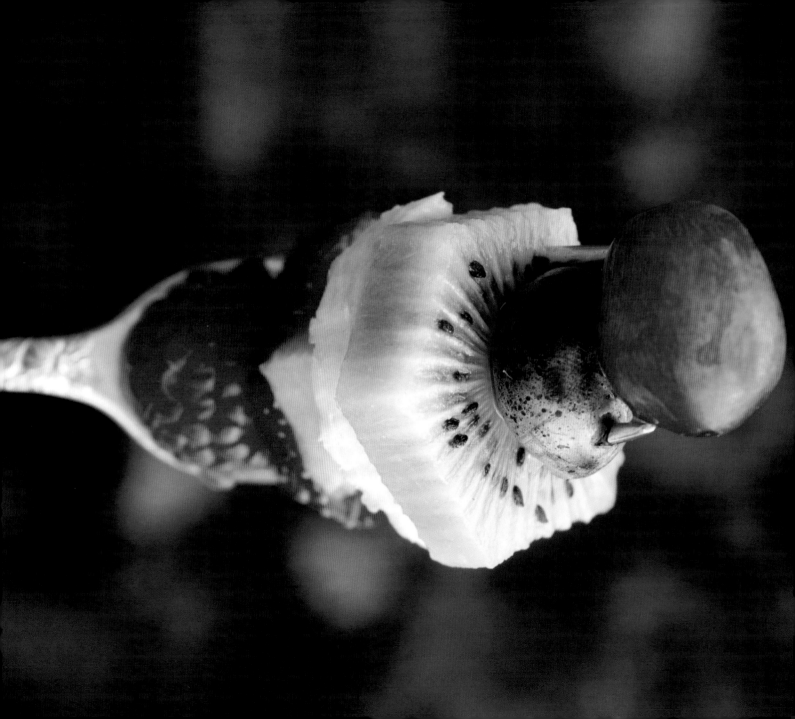

CHAKRA FRUIT SALAD *(v)*

"It's so beautifully arranged on the plate—you know someone's fingers have been all over it." JULIA CHILD

Our Chakra Fruit Salad represents the seven chakra colors found in our bodies (see Chakra Vegetable Slaw recipe on page 126 for more on chakras). It is delicious with our Fantasy Fruit dressing drizzled on top. Serves 8–10.

½ cup *Fantasy Fruit dressing* (see recipe on page 152)

1 cup raspberries
1 cup small strawberries (stems removed)
1 cup cantaloupe (cut into ¾-inch cubes)
1 cup banana (cut into ½-inch slices)
1 cup kiwi (cut into half moon slices)
1 cup blueberries (stems removed)
1 cup purple seedless grapes (stems removed)

1. Prepare dressing.
2. Prepare fruit and arrange individually by type in rows to form a "rainbow" of fruit starting with purple at the top of the plate.
3. Dress fruit immediately before serving or serve dressing on the side in individual bowls.
4. Serve and delight!

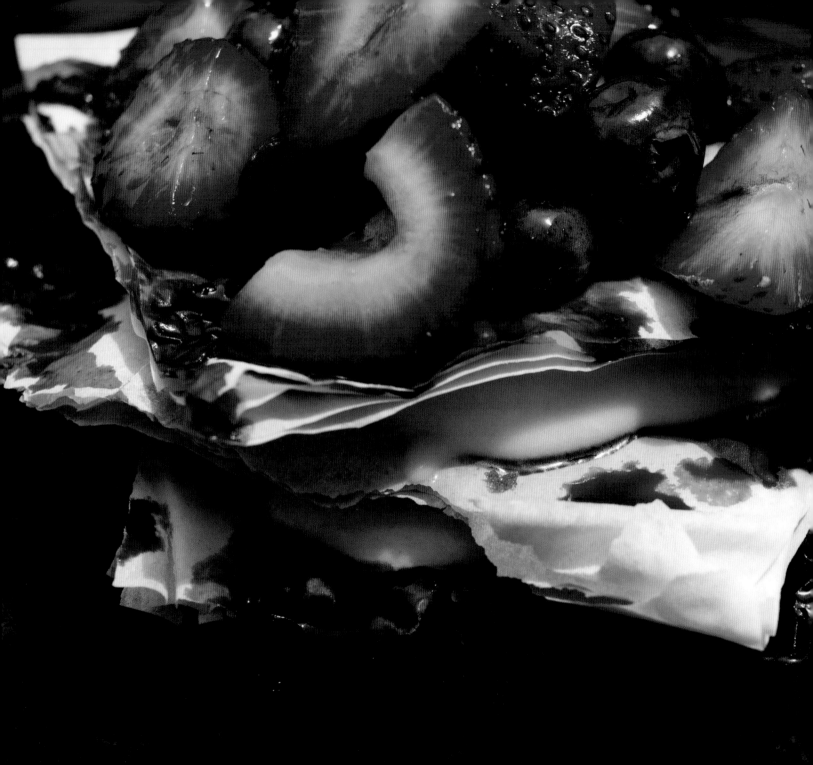

NAMASTE NAPOLEONS (v)

We often offer "Namaste" at the end of our yoga classes. Though it is so widely used, many people do not know the meaning of the word. In fact, for a while, Kristen's dad thought people were saying, "Have a nice day . . . " and her daughter, four years old, says, "Momaste" (and we couldn't correct that!). Though these variations are lovely, the gesture Namaste is truly an acknowledgment of the soul in one by the soul in another. Nama = bow, as = I, and te = you. Thus, the English translation is "I bow to you." So, with love in our hearts, we present these Namaste Napoleons to you. Serves 4.

Blueberry Compote
2 cups frozen blueberries
3T water
¼ cup brown sugar
1T lemon juice
1T fresh tarragon (chopped)

½ cup maple syrup
2 tsp. vanilla extract

36 sheets of Filo pastry
2T olive oil (in mister)
2T brown sugar

Coconut Whipped Cream
1 16 oz. refrigerated (overnight) unshaken can of
    coconut milk (liquid poured off)

Topping
1 cup fresh blueberries
1 cup fresh strawberries (de-stemmed and sliced)

1. Preheat oven to 400°F.
2. Prepare *Blueberry Compote* by combining ingredients in a medium saucepan over low-medium heat. Bring ingredients to a simmer and cook for about 10 minutes, stirring frequently. Remove from heat. Allow to cool to room temperature.
3. Prepare *Coconut Whipped Cream*. Place cold coconut solid, maple syrup, and vanilla in a cold, medium mixing bowl. Using a hand mixer, whip ingredients together until it forms a whipped cream–like consistency. Set in refrigerator until use.
4. Prepare fresh fruit by combining blueberries and strawberry slices.
5. Mist 12 stacks of three 4 x 4 inch sheets of Filo pastry equally with olive oil and equally sprinkle with brown sugar. Toast Filo stacks in batches on a baking sheet in oven for about 2 minutes on each side or until golden brown. Set aside.
6. Begin layering Napoleons. Start with one 3-sheet stack of baked Filo. Top with 2 tablespoons of *Coconut Whipped Cream, then 3* tablespoons of *Blueberry Compote.* Repeat that layering process one more time. Top *Napoleons* with a third stack of Filo. Top with 1 tablespoon of whipped cream and ½ cup of fresh berries. Repeat 4 times to make 4 individual *Namaste Napoleons.*
7. Serve and enjoy immediately.

ANJALI MUDRA
HAND GESTURE WITH NAMASTE OR PRAYER SEAL

supports gratitude, encourages stillness, grounding, uplifting

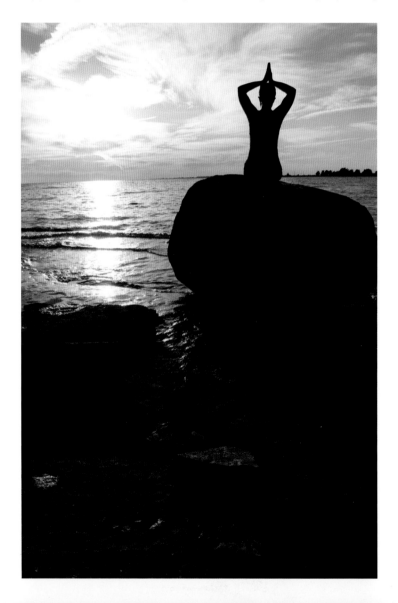

PURPOSE

"For those who have an intense urge for Spirit and wisdom, it sits near them, waiting."
PATANJALI, *THE YOGA SUTRAS OF PATANJALI*

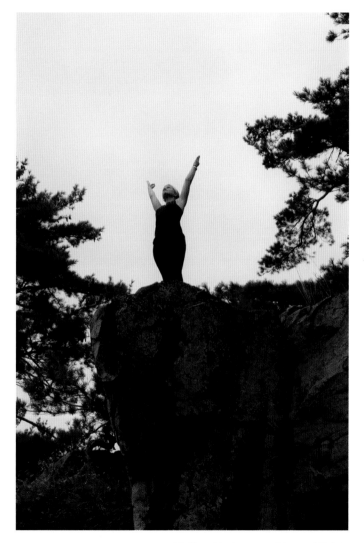

Urdhva Hastasana • Upward Salute

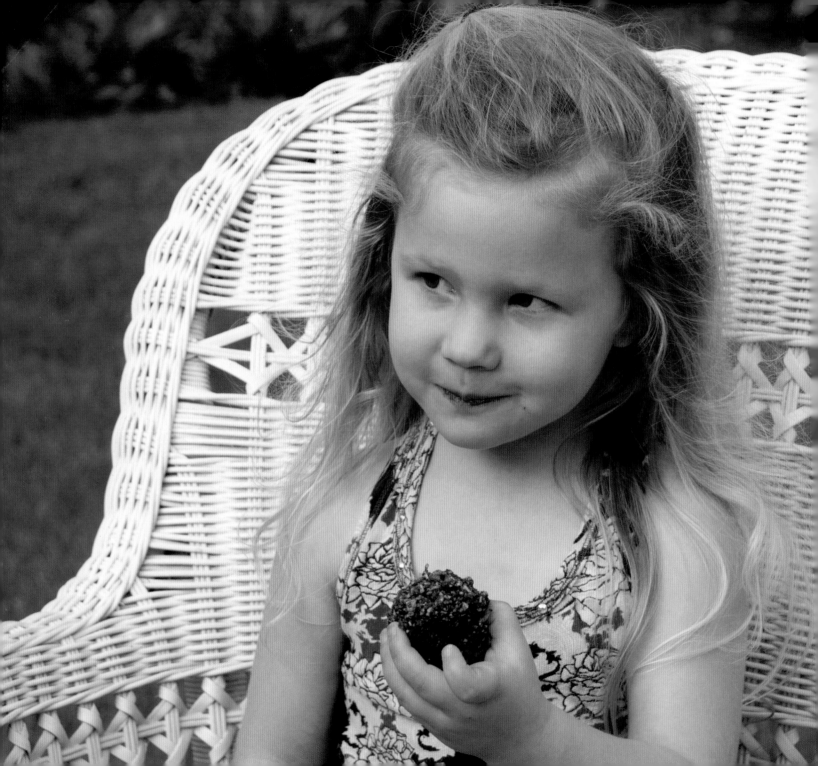

GRACE'S NO-BAKES (v)

This is a twist on classic no-bake cookie recipes. Our recipe is a bit healthier than the traditional recipe, vegan, and a fan-favorite of Kristen's daughter, Grace. These cookies are so good that we felt compelled to try the recipe again, for the second time, the day after our initial recipe trial. We're still not sure how the first batch of cookies disappeared so quickly! Makes about 20 cookies. (These cookies may be stored in the refrigerator in an airtight container for up to 4 days.)

2 cups quick cooking oats
1 cup unsweetened coconut flakes
½ cup chocolate chips (dairy free)
½ cup raw almonds (crushed)
Himalayan salt coarsely ground (to taste)
½ cup almond butter
½ cup coconut solids from refrigerated (overnight) unshaken can of coconut milk (liquid poured off)
½ cup brown sugar (packed)
2T dark cocoa powder
½ tsp. pure vanilla

1. In a large mixing bowl combine oats, coconut flakes, chocolate chips, raw almonds, and salt.
2. Stir almond butter, coconut solids, brown sugar, and cocoa powder in a saucepan over low-medium heat until sugar and cocoa are dissolved.
3. Take mixture off of heat and add in vanilla.
4. Pour cocoa mixture over oat mixture and combine.
5. Using two spoons or an ice cream scoop, form about 2 tablespoons of batter into abstract rounds and drop onto a parchment paper–lined baking sheet. Place cookies in the refrigerator until they are set, or for at least 1 hour.
6. Serve and delight!

GRACE

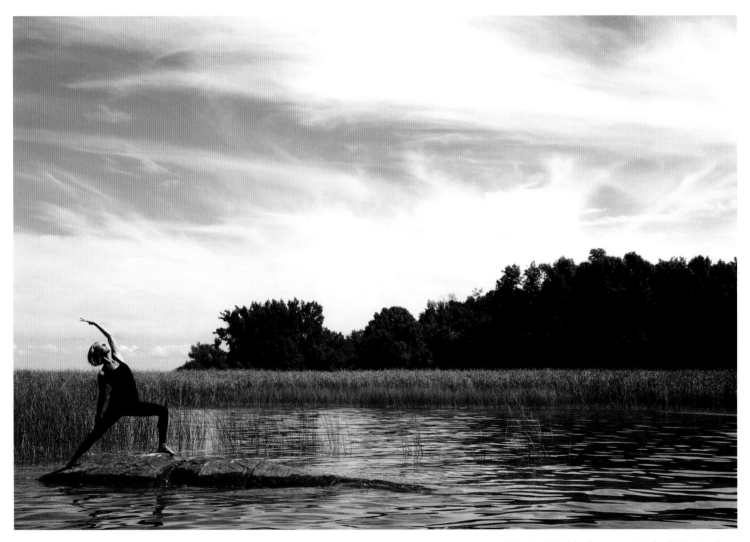

Viparita Virabhadrasana • Exalted Warrior Pose

POWER

People with high-paying or high-profile jobs are often perceived to have power. Money or fame, however, cannot provide us with the same level of power that comes from inner contentment, non-harming (ahimsa), compassion, and grace. True power comes from belief of your path and what you possess from within.

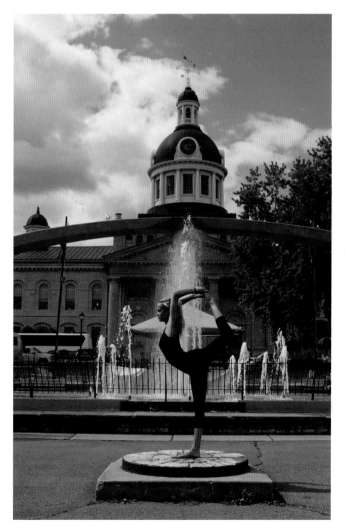

Natarajasana III • Advanced King Dancer

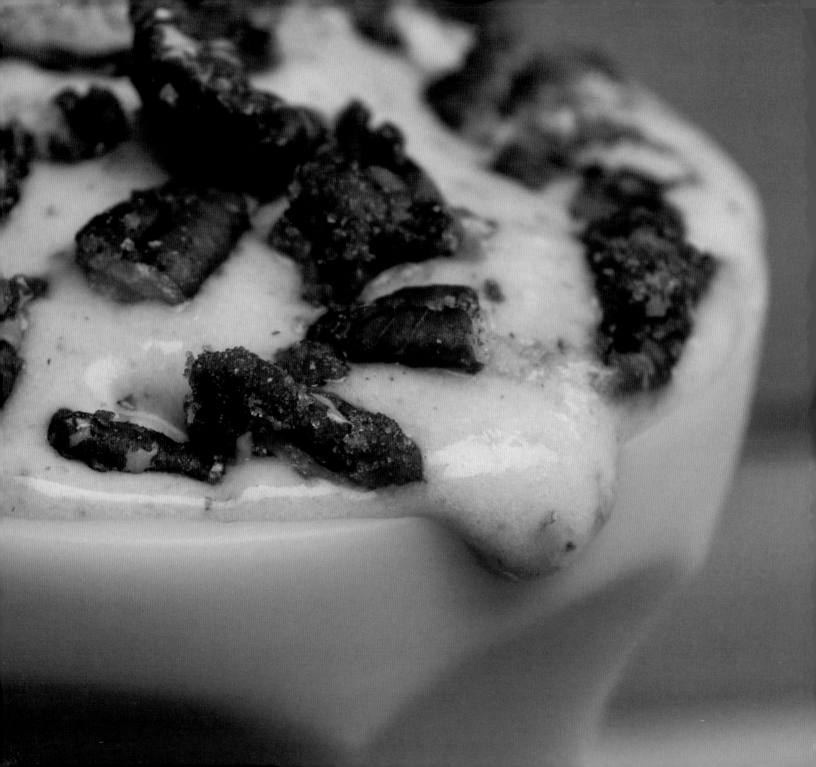

BANANA BLISS *(v)*

If there's such a thing as bliss-in-a-cup, this is it! Our Banana Bliss desserts are refreshing and absolutely delightful! Plus, bananas contain potassium, which reduces swelling, increases energy, strengthens our nervous system, and improves digestion. Serves 4–8.

> 1 cup chopped toasted nuts (walnuts, pecans, or combination)
> 2T brown sugar
> 3 frozen, peeled bananas
> 2T almond milk
> 1 16 oz. refrigerated (overnight) unshaken can of coconut milk (liquid poured off)
> 1 tsp. vanilla extract

1. Toast nuts in a medium skillet over low-medium heat, adding salt to taste throughout the process, until golden brown and fragrant. Stir in brown sugar and cook for another 1 to 2 minutes, or until sugar is dissolved. Remove from heat and place in refrigerator.
2. Combine bananas, almond milk, coconut solids, and vanilla in food processor until just combined. Add cool nuts and pulse slightly.
3. Serve immediately in individual glasses. Enjoy!

BLISS

"Follow your bliss and the universe will open doors for you where there were only walls."
JOSEPH CAMPBELL

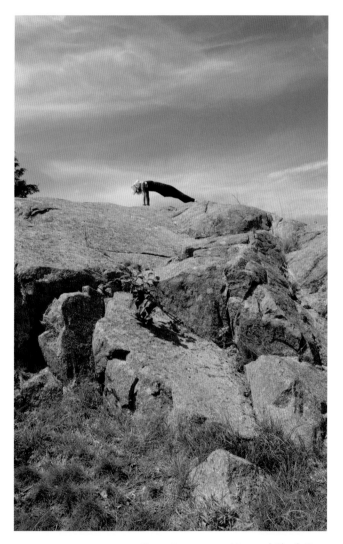

Purvottanasana • Upward Plank Pose

DREAM

"Dreams are illustrations . . . from the book your soul is writing about you."
MARSHA NORMAN

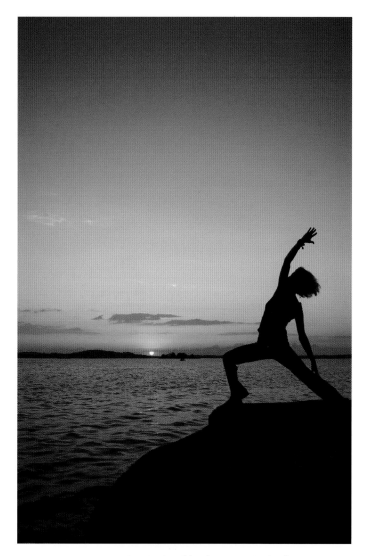

Viparita Virabhadrasana • Exalted Warrior Pose

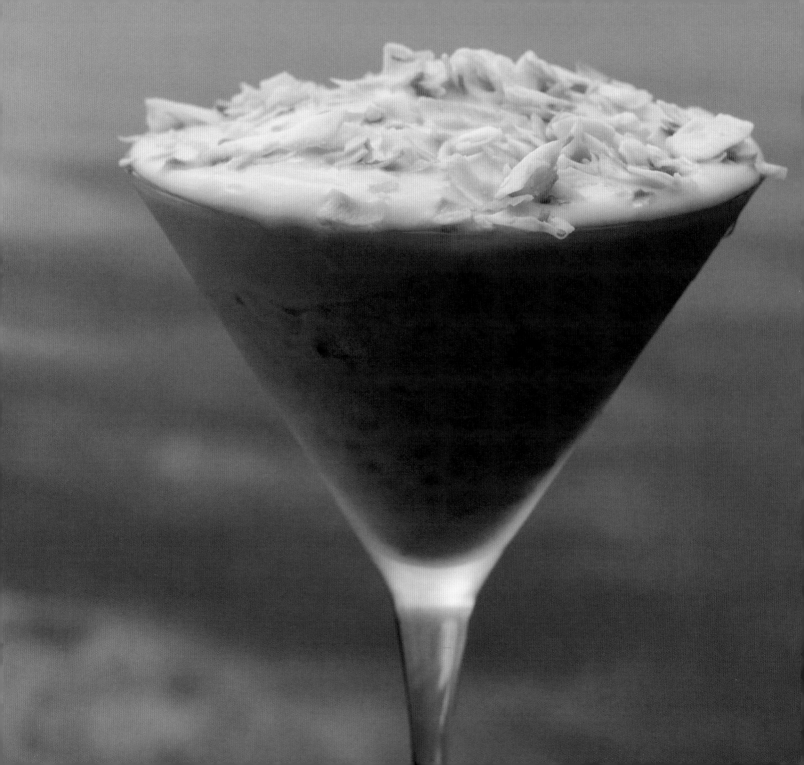

COCONUT CREAM DREAMS *(v)(r)*

"To sleep, perchance to dream . . ." Sleep is a very important ingredient for living a healthy life. And with sleep, we dream. Our dreams have the ability to reveal to us the truths of our inner emotions. They may be fantasy-filled, encouraging, inspiring, or even a little scary. When we pay attention to our dreams, they may help to guide us in a wonderful, and possibly, more honest direction. Our Coconut Cream Dreams are ridiculously dreamy. You don't need a lot of this dessert to be satiated. Variation: Enjoy the coconut raw for a completely raw variation of this dish. Enjoy and surrender. Serves 8–12.

Delight Base
1 cup unsweetened coconut (plus ¼ cup for topping)
1 cup whole dates (pitted)
1 ½ cups raw cashews
1 16 oz. refrigerated (overnight) can of coconut milk
1 tsp. vanilla extract

Coconut Whipped Cream
1 16 oz. refrigerated (overnight) unshaken can of coconut milk (liquid poured off)
½ cup maple syrup
2 tsp. pure vanilla extract

1. Toast unsweetened coconut in a medium skillet over low-medium heat until slightly golden brown. Remove from heat and set aside.
2. Prepare *Delight Base* by combining 1 cup toasted coconut, dates, cashews, coconut milk, and vanilla in a food processor. Pour *Base* directly into individual serving dishes (to desired amount).
3. Prepare *Coconut Whipped Cream*. Place cold coconut solid, maple syrup, and vanilla in a cold, medium mixing bowl. Using a hand mixer, whip ingredients together until it becomes a whipped cream–like consistency. Place equally on top of individual serving dishes and refrigerate until serving.
4. Before serving, top with remaining toasted coconut.

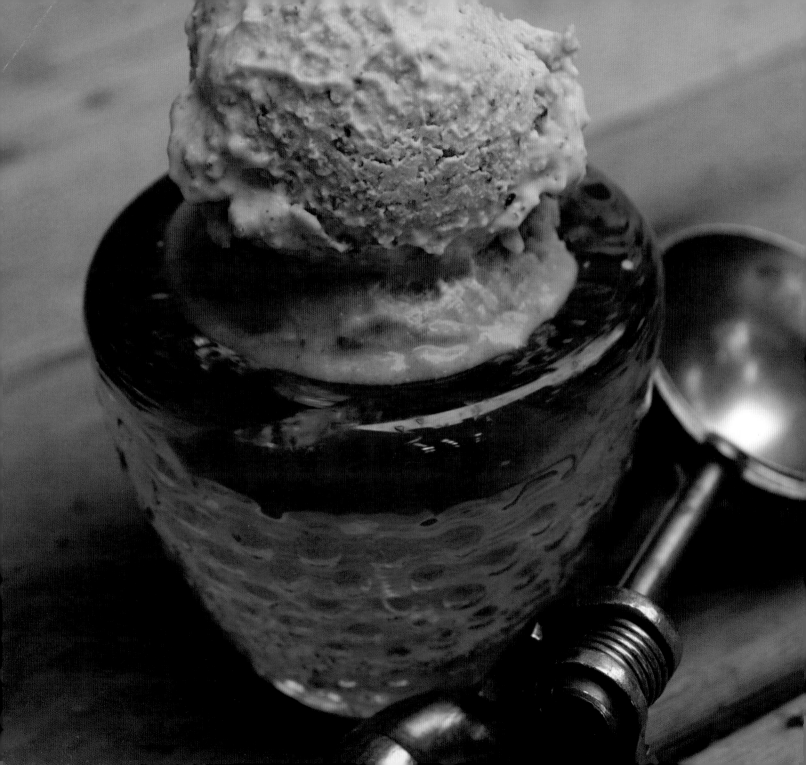

PERFECTLY IMPERFECT PUMKIN PIE ICE CREAM (v)

This is yet another circumstance where we were going for one thing and found another (and we're happy we did)! Our no-bake pumpkin pie recipe (not included in this book for good reasons) turned out to be totally imperfect, but the flavors were perfectly amazing. Thus, what was initially a pie recipe transformed beautifully into an ice cream! Best yet, it's vegan! Serves 12.

16 oz. canned pumpkin
½ cup almond milk
2 16 oz. refrigerated (overnight) unshaken cans of
  coconut milk (liquid poured off)
1 cup 100% pure maple syrup
2 tsp. vanilla extract

½ tsp. ground ginger
½ tsp. ground cinnamon
¼ tsp. ground nutmeg
½ cup raw pecans
½ cup raw almonds

1. Combine ingredients in a food processor until mixture reaches uniform consistency.
2. Place into ice cream machine and allow to churn for about 25–30 minutes or until it reaches desired consistency. Serve or place in your freezer in an airtight storage container for 2 hours for harder ice cream.

PEACEFUL PISTACHIO FROZEN YOGURT

"World peace must develop from inner peace. Peace is not just mere absence of violence. Peace is, I think, the manifestation of human compassion." HIS HOLINESS THE XIV DALAI LAMA

This frozen yogurt recipe is splendidly decadent. Pistachios have been shown to aid in weight management and healthy heart functioning. Serves 6–8.

1 cup shelled unsalted pistachios
1 16 oz. refrigerated (overnight) unshaken can of coconut milk (liquid poured off)
2 tsp. vanilla extract
10 oz. strained Greek honey yogurt
1T agave nectar
Himalayan salt finely ground (to taste)

1. Combine ingredients in a food processor.
2. Place into ice cream machine and allow to churn for about 25–30 minutes or until it reaches desired consistency. Serve or place in freezer in an airtight storage container for 2 hours for harder frozen yogurt.

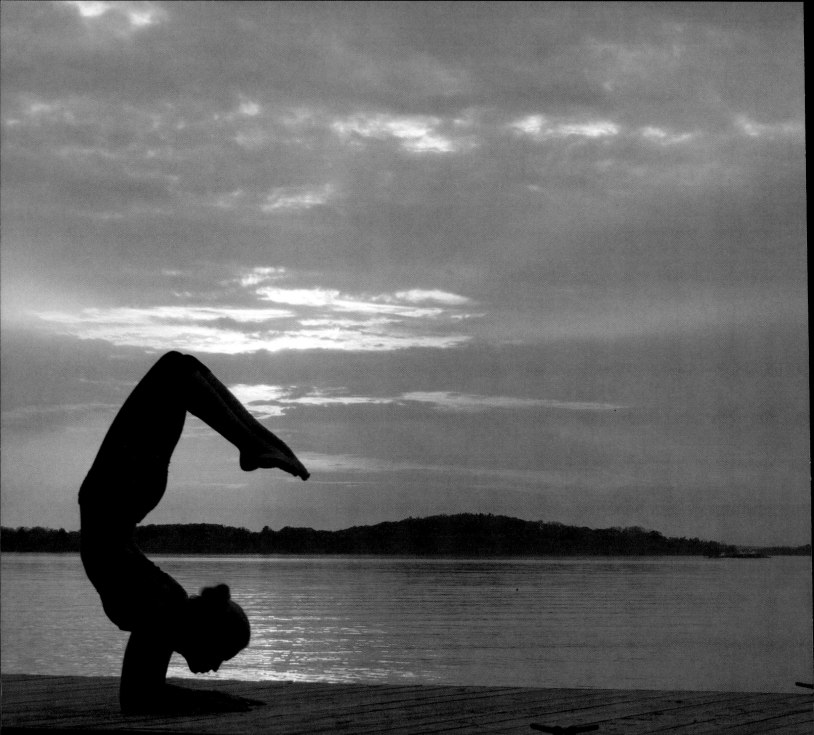

FOUNTAINS OF YOUTH

AWARENESS

*"There are only two ways to live your life. One is as though nothing is a miracle.
The other is as though everything is a miracle."*
ALBERT EINSTEIN

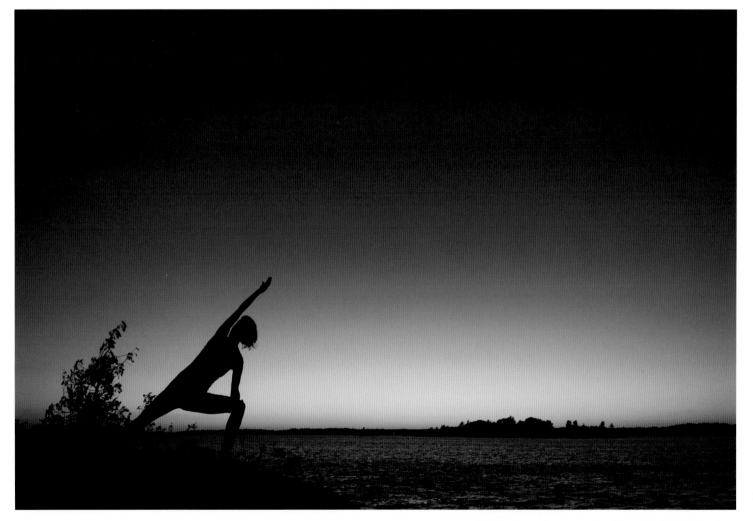

Utthita Parsvakonasana I • Extended Side Angle Pose

SALAMBA SARVANGASANA
SUPPORTED SHOULDERSTAND

soothing, relaxing, "queen of all poses"
and "fountain of youth"

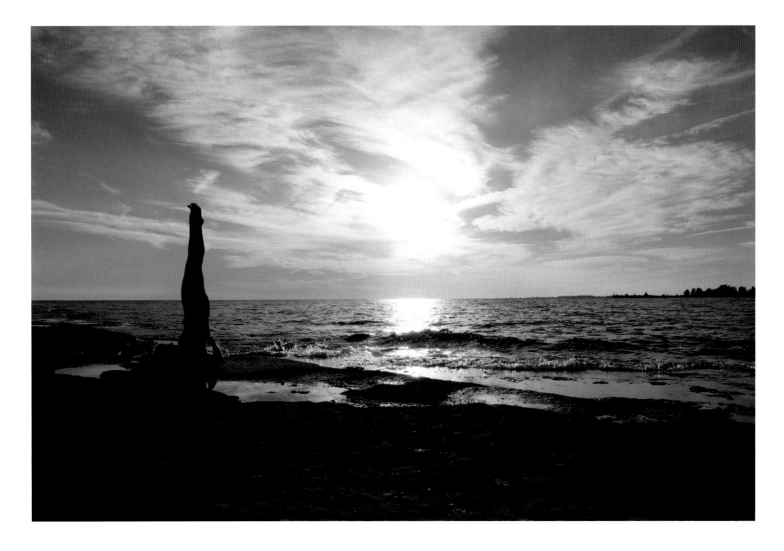

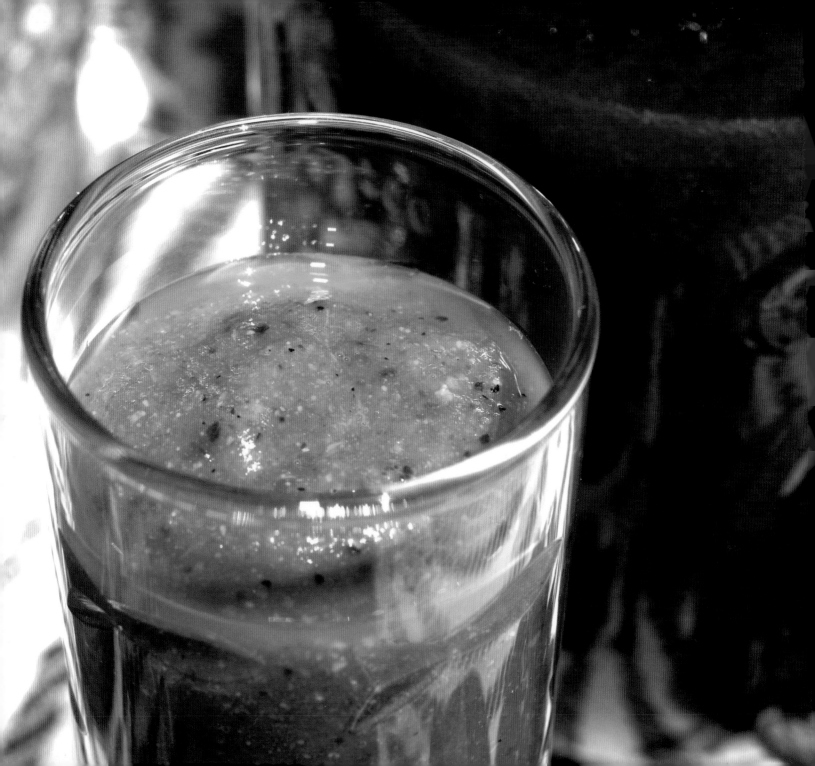

BIRD OF PARADISE PIÑA COLADA *(v)(r)*

As we find when moving into Bird of Paradise pose, the beauty lies at the fine line between effort and ease. Here we are comfortable with our actions and inactions. Here we blossom! Our shakes, juices, and water drinks are big on taste and benefits of the mind and body. Our Bird of Paradise Piña Colada smoothie contains coconut solids and coconut water. Many Asian and Pacific populations call the coconut palm "The Tree of Life," as they consider it to be the cure for illness as well as a great food source; it is rich in fiber, vitamins, and minerals. Serves 2.

2T coconut solids from refrigerated (overnight) unshaken can of coconut milk (liquid poured off)
1 cup coconut water
½ frozen, peeled banana
1 cup fresh mango
1 ½ cups fresh pineapple
½ cup ice
Agave nectar to taste (optional)

Combine all ingredients in a blender. Serve.

KEY LIME SPLIT *(v)(r)*

This Key Lime Split smoothie is totally refreshing. Nutrient-dense coconut combined with fresh fruits and zesty key limes create a well-balanced drink. Key limes are full of one of nature's best antioxidants, Vitamin C. All of our smoothies, shakes, and juices are wonderful because they are filling and good for us; essentially, they are blended, satiating snacks or meals. Serves 2.

2T coconut solids from refrigerated (overnight) unshaken can of coconut milk (liquid poured off)
1T coconut water
2T agave nectar
½ frozen, peeled banana
½ cup fresh pineapple
Juice from two key limes (regular limes may be substituted)
1 cup ice

Combine all ingredients in a blender. Serve.

SVARGA DVIJASANA
BIRD OF PARADISE

opens hips, provides balance

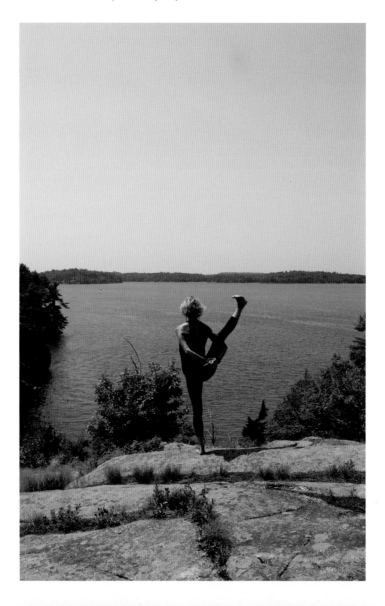

URDHVA PRASARITA EKA PADASANA
STANDING SPLIT

calming, emotionally supportive, improves concentration

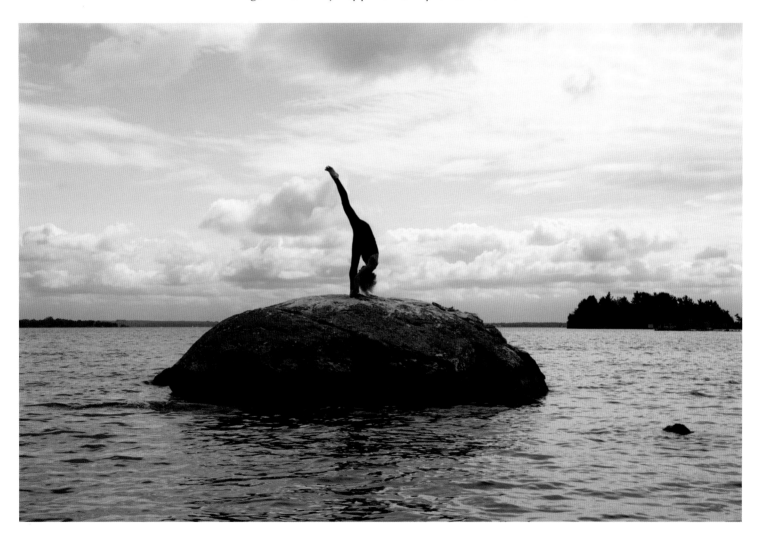

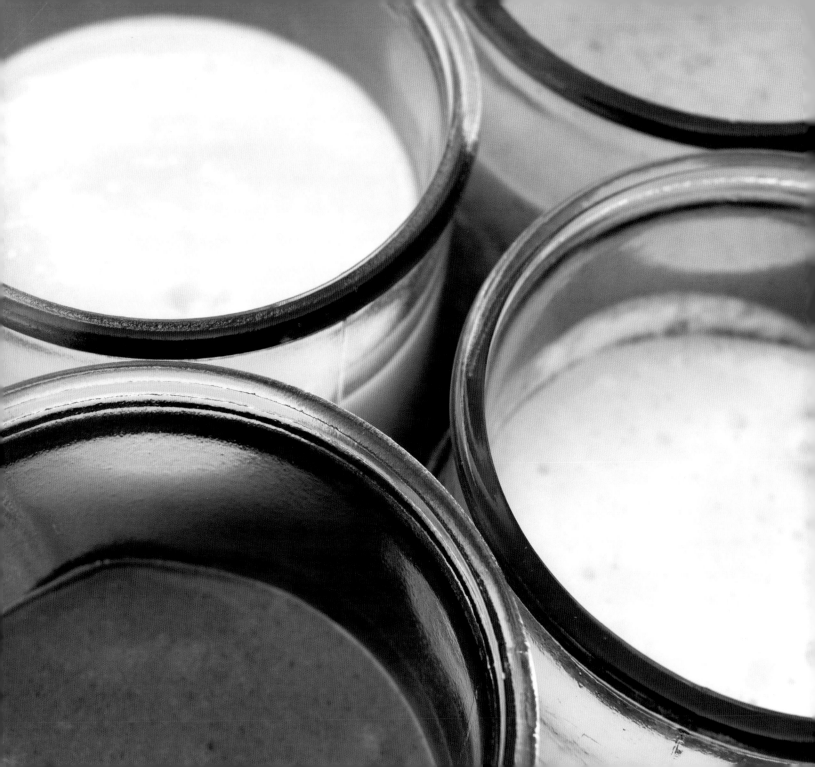

MONKEYING AROUND (v)

Set the child in you free with our Monkeying Around shake. Enjoy the freedom of being! Almonds are a great source of protein and fiber. We are big fans of nut spreads—almond butter, cashew butter and sunflower butter, are three of our favorites. Serves 2.

1½ cups almond milk
3 frozen, peeled bananas
½ tsp. ground cinnamon
½ cup of almond butter
1T agave nectar
Himalayan salt coarsely ground (to taste)

Combine all ingredients in a blender. Serve.

DIVINE DARK CHOCOLATE GINGERBREAD CAKE (v)

Yum, yum, yum! Our Divine Dark Chocolate Gingerbread Cake shake is out of this world. This beverage would make a wake-up-worthy breakfast treat. Serves 2.

2T coconut solids from refrigerated (overnight) unshaken can of coconut milk (liquid poured off)
½ cup almond milk
1 frozen, peeled banana
1T dark cocoa powder
1 tsp. ground ginger
½ cup of almond butter
3T pure maple syrup
Himalayan salt coarsely ground (to taste)

Combine all ingredients in a blender. Serve.

HANUMANASANA
MONKEY GOD POSTURE

calming, stretching,
invigorating

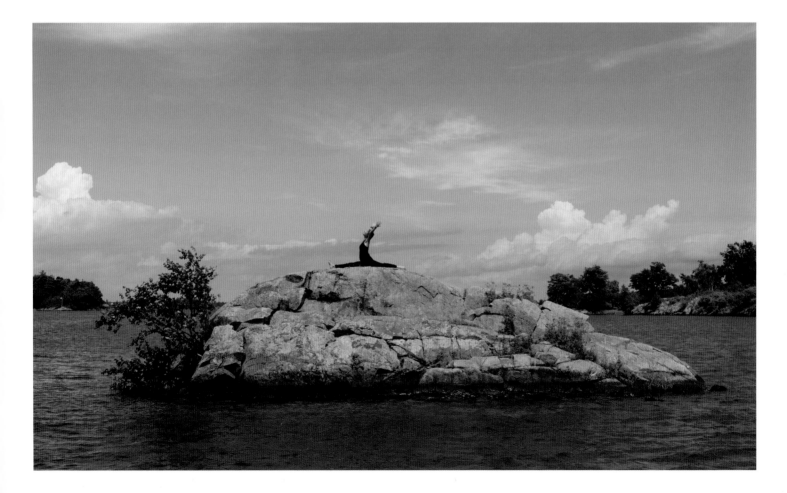

NATURE

"Life's a river, you gotta go where it takes you."
SHIVA REA

Pancha mahabhuta is a basic concept of Ayurveda (Ayur = Life, Veda = Knowledge), an ancient, time-honored practice of natural medicine healing that originated in India. The pancha mahabhuta theory outlines that there are "five great elements"—earth, water, fire, air, and space—that govern the balance of our bodies and environments. The theory also suggests that upon death all five elements of the human body remain in nature, thereby balancing the natural cycle.

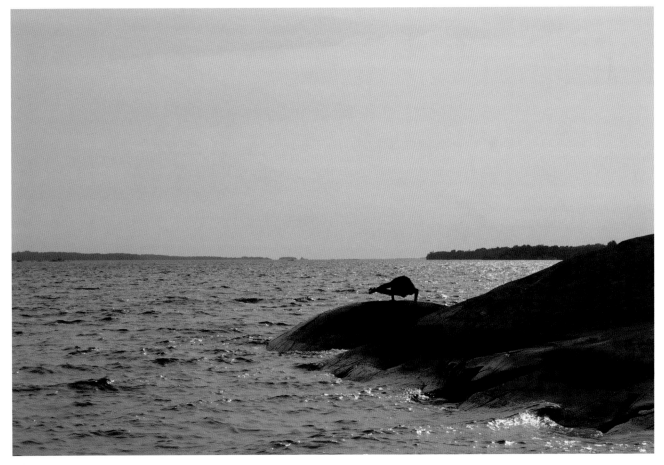

Astavakrasana • Eight Angle Pose

HUMILITY

"The more I learn, the more I realize how much I don't know."
ALBERT EINSTEIN

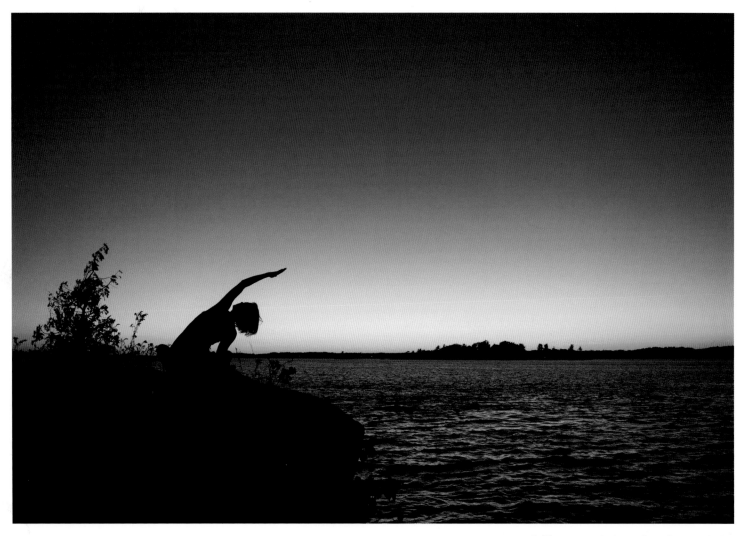

Sukhasana variation • Easy Pose variation

SAVASANA
CORPSE POSE

calms, relaxes, promotes regular breathing, allows mind to find stillness

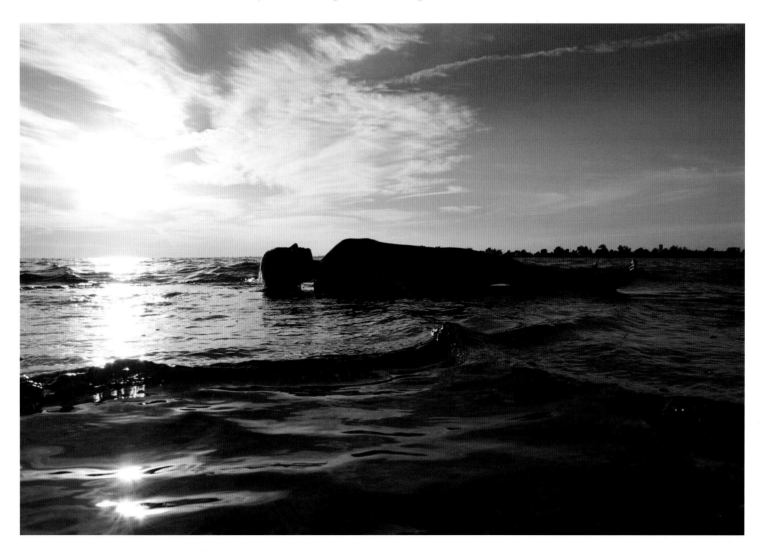

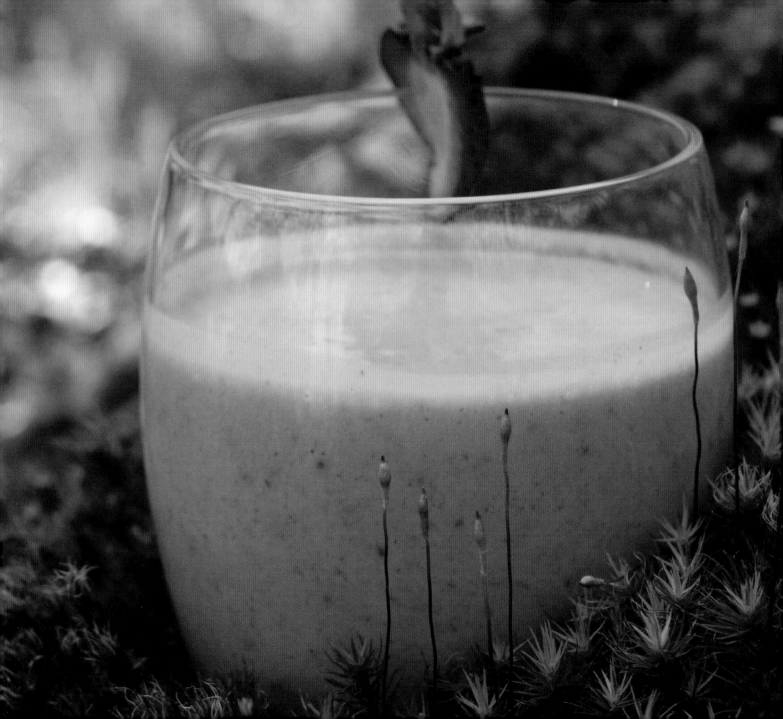

STRAWBERRY SAVASANA

The simple truth is that when we eat more fresh fruits and vegetables and fewer processed foods, we become healthier. Strawberries contain a plethora of very powerful antioxidants that help to counter the effects of free radicals. They also contain folic acid, which may aid in healthy pregnancies. Our Strawberry Savasana smoothie is delicious and child-approved. Serves 2–4.

    1 cup fresh strawberries
    1 cup frozen strawberries
    ½ cup mango
    1 frozen, peeled banana
    1 cup strained honey yogurt
    1T agave nectar
    ½ cup coconut water
    Himalayan salt coarsely ground (to taste)

    Combine all ingredients in a blender. Serve.

CELEBRATE

"The more you praise and celebrate your life, the more there is in life to celebrate."
OPRAH WINFREY

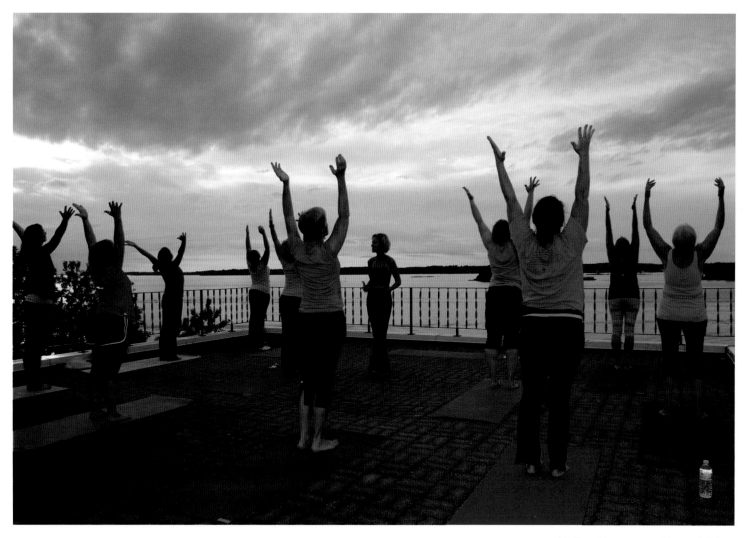

Urdhva Hastasana • Upward Salute

PLAY

As children, play, openness, fearlessness, and laughter are part of our true nature. As adults, living freely in the moment and accepting those things we can no longer change provides opportunity to feel that joy we all originally, and effortlessly, celebrated.

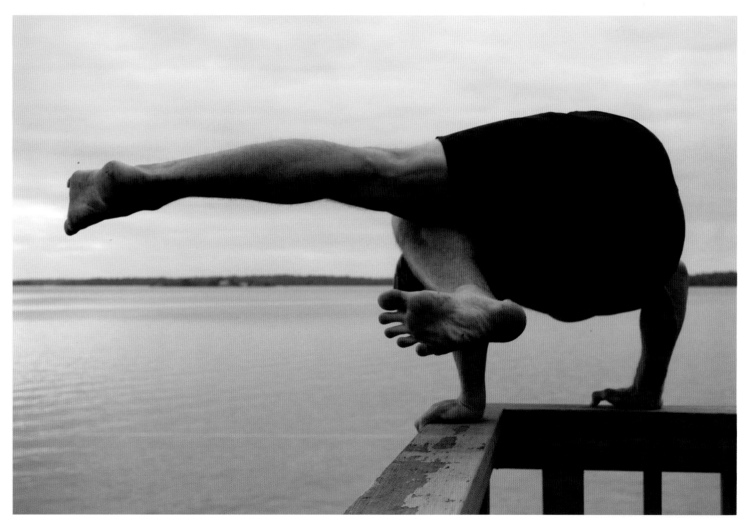

Parsva Bakasana • Side Crow

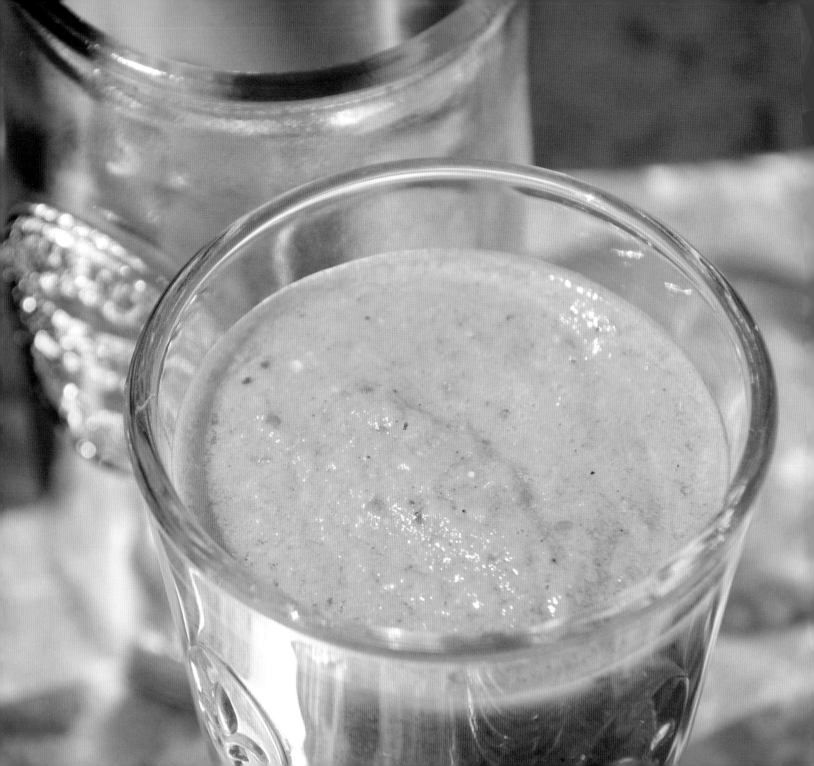

FLYING CARROT

We cannot say enough about the "amazingness" of carrots. Carrots contain the antioxidant beta-carotene and are an excellent source of Vitamin A, helping us to glow from the inside out. Our Flying Carrot juice combines a perfect combination of savory and sweet flavors. Serves 2.

2 carrots
¼ banana (peeled)
½ cup soy milk
¼ cup honey yogurt
1T fresh ginger

Combine all ingredients in a blender. Serve.

BLOODY MERRY (a.k.a. HAIR OF THE DOG) *(v)*

Our Bloody Merry (a.k.a. Hair of the Dog) juice is perfect for when we're feeling under the weather, dehydrated, or just want a rejuvenating drink. We include horseradish in this juice because it adds a great kick and also contains cancer-fighting compounds called glucosinolates. Serves 2.

4 large tomatoes (seeded)
2 stalks celery (leaves removed)
1T fresh ginger
1 medium garlic clove
1T fresh horseradish
2T lemon juice
1 tsp. lemon flaxseed oil
1 tsp. tamari
Dash of cayenne
Dash of turmeric
Dash of celery salt
Pepper coarsely ground (to taste)

Combine ingredients in a blender. Serve.

EKA PADA GALAVASANA
FLYING CROW

strengthening, balancing, powerful

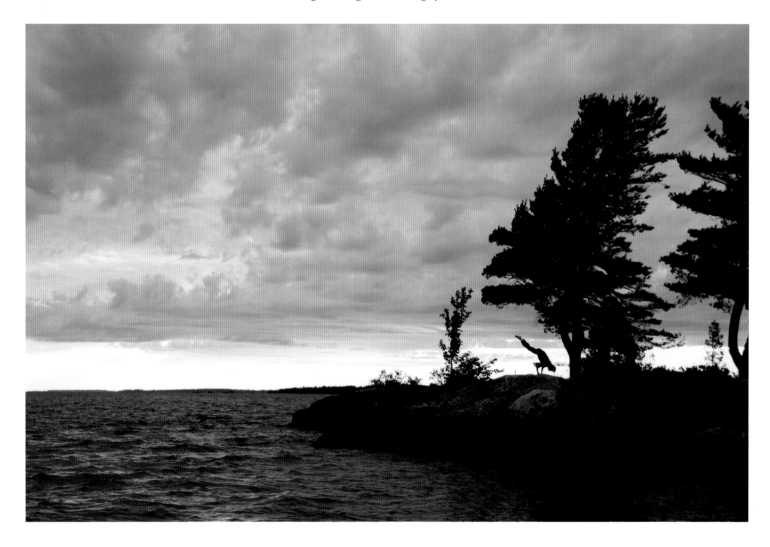

URDHVA MUKHA SVANASANA
UPWARD FACING DOG POSE

strengthens spine, stimulates organs, opens heart center

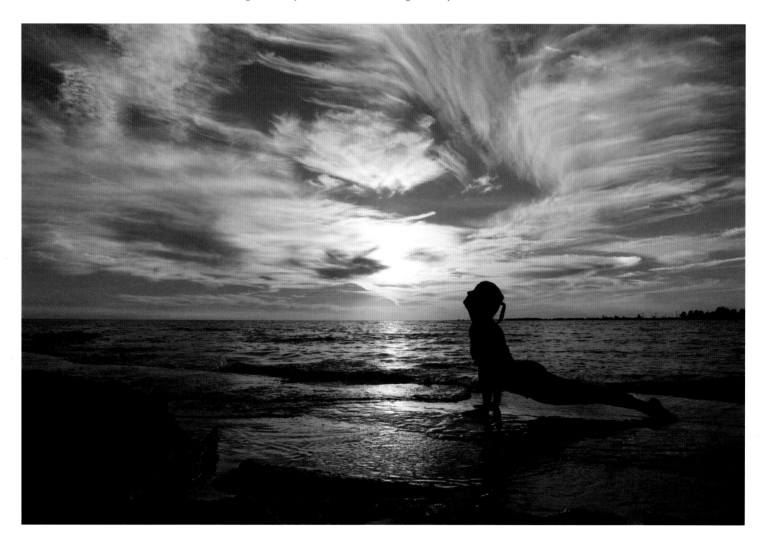

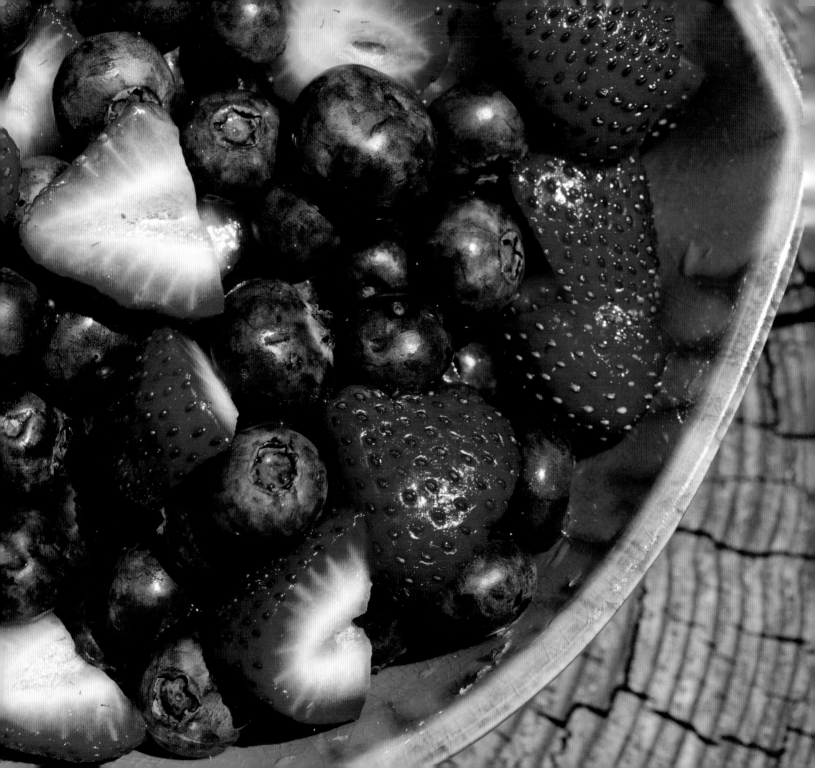

BLUEBERRY BEET BAKASANA *(v)(r)*

Juices provide a healthful, satisfying way to consume a variety of raw fruits and vegetables. Blueberries are repeatedly touted for having one of the highest antioxidant capacities. They also offer potential benefits for the nervous system and brain health. Our Blueberry Beet Bakasana is a delicious, nutritious, vibrant-colored juice. Serves 2.

1 cup blueberries
1 large beet (peeled)
½ apple
1 kiwi (peeled)
2 stalks of celery
2T coconut water

Combine all ingredients in a blender. Serve.

THAI DANCER *(v)(r)*

When we concentrate on maintaining deep and steady breathing in yoga as well as treating our poses and transitions as postures, we begin to float or even dance throughout our practices. Our Thai Dancer juice is inspired by Thai cooking flavors and packs a sweet and spicy punch. We think this makes a great mid-afternoon juice. Serves 1.

1 cup kale
¼ cup cilantro leaves
1T mint leaves
¼ Serrano chili pepper
½ cup fresh pineapple chunks
2T lime juice

Combine all ingredients in a blender. Serve chilled.

BAKASANA
CROW

*strengthening, helps to develop
concentration and balance*

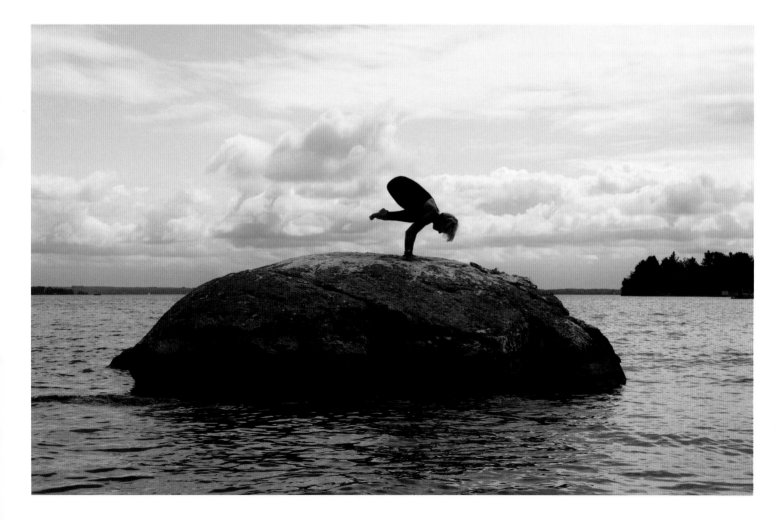

EXPLORE

"Deep within lies a real and everlasting joy. A human being is born to dive deep into the stream of life, find the hidden treasure, and attain eternal fulfillment."
SRIMAD BHAGAVATAM

Take your practice off your mat, through the kitchen, and into the world.

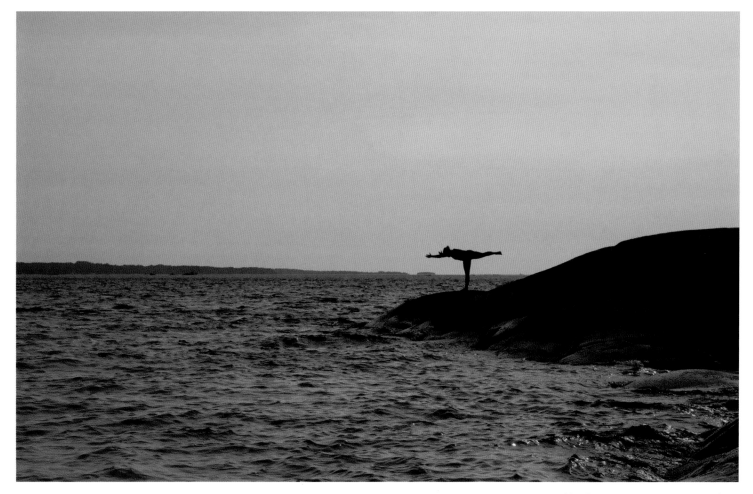

Virabhadrasana III • Warrior Pose Three

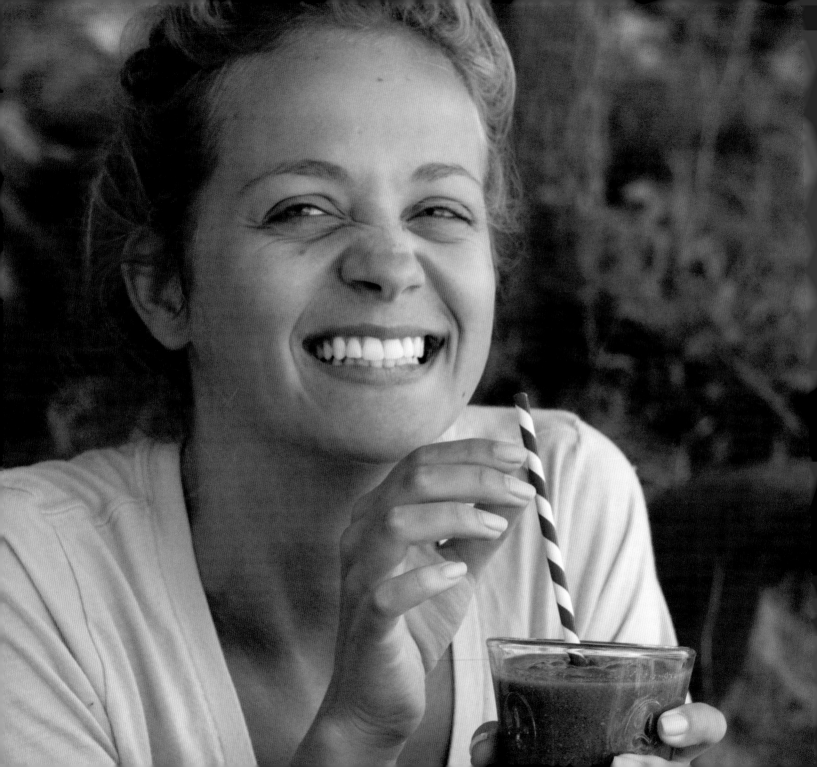

GOOD MORNING, GODDESS! *(v)(r)*

Our Good Morning, Goddess! juice is packed with fiber-rich, dark leafy greens and naturally sweet fruits. This juice was designed to bring out our inner goddess even on our most un-goddess-like mornings. Drink up and glow from the inside out! Serves 1.

1 cup spinach
½ cup cucumber
1 kiwi (peeled)
1 pear (cored)

Combine all ingredients in a blender. Serve.

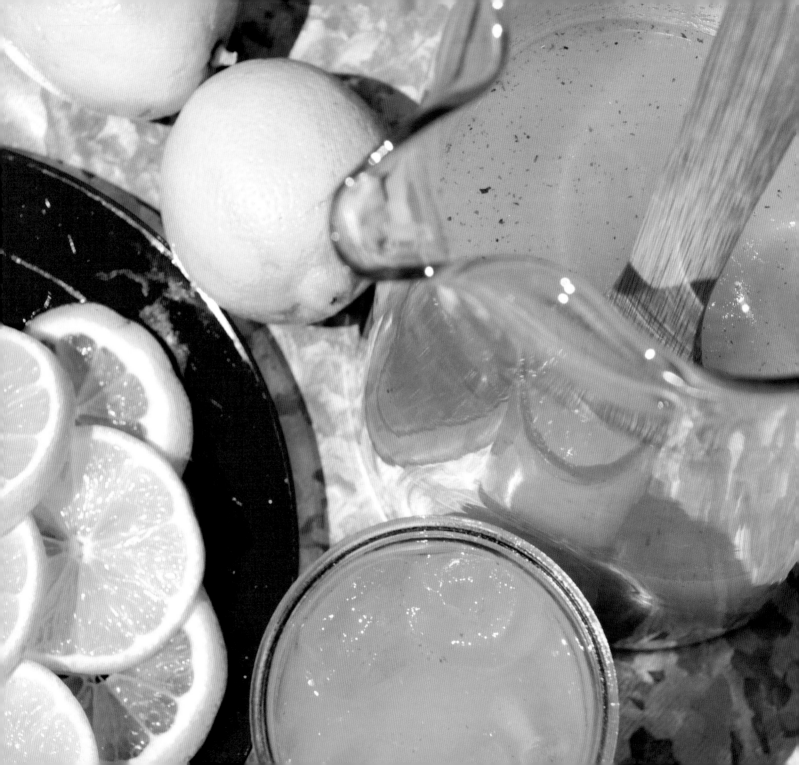

COCONUT CAMEL LEMONADE *(v)(r)*

Coconut water has gained mainstream popularity over the last few years. It contains more calcium, potassium, and magnesium than most juices. It is one of the best hydrators, helping us to restore our muscles during and after our practices. The addition of lemon and ginger to this water gives it an extra nutritional boost as well as strong citrus flavor. This is a raw, thirst-quenching lemonade-style drink. Serves 2–4.

½ cup lemon juice
1 tsp. fresh ginger
1T mint leaves
1 cup coconut water
1 cup water
2T agave nectar (or to taste)
1T fresh mint.

Optional Garnishes
Mint leaves
Lemon slices

1. Combine all ingredients in a blender.
2. Serve over ice and garnish as desired.

ARDHA USTRASANA
HALF CAMEL POSTURE

improves posture, helps to balance chakras, relieves lower back pain

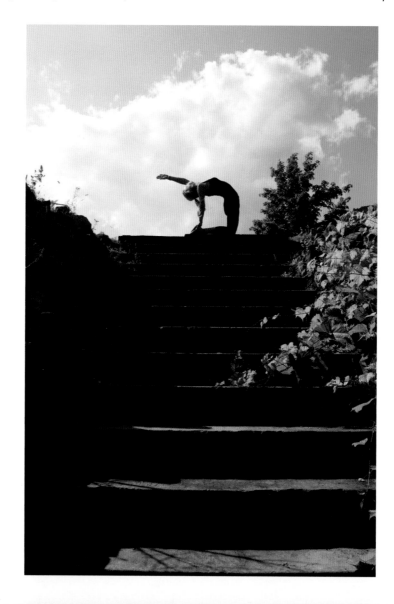

NATARAJASANA III
ADVANCED KING DANCER

improves balance, opens heart center, stretches shoulders

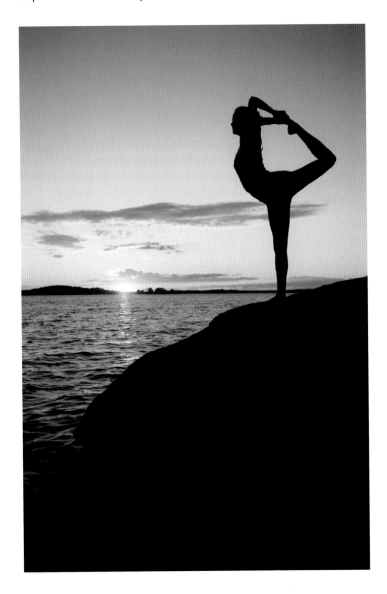

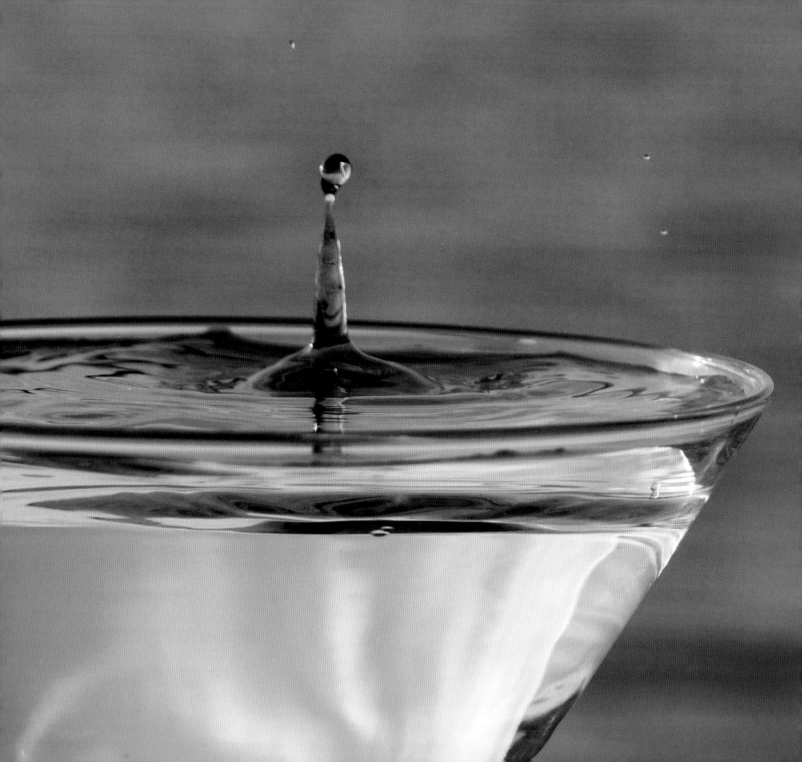

WATER TABLE (WITH FOOD GRADE ESSENTIAL OILS) *(v)(r)*

Food grade essential oils boast many more uses than aromatic amazement. They may offer calming, energizing, and other effects on the mind, body, and inner spirit. Extracted from flowers, trees, and roots, they are nature's gifts. We like to drink 10 8-ounce glasses of water a day to stay well hydrated. Once a day, we often include a drop of food grade essential oil in our water. Below are some of our favorites:

LEMON OIL is energizing and uplifting and serves as an antioxidant

LIME OIL may boost clarity, creativity, and also support a healthy immune system

PEPPERMINT OIL is fresh, energizing, invigorating, helps to combat fatigue, and may promote healthy respiratory function

HEALING

Acupuncture, aromatherapy, Ayurvedic medicine, homeopathy, massage, meditation, naturopathic therapy, Reiki, reflexology, and yoga are all ancient, time-tested practices for promoting whole health—wellness of the mind, body, and inner spirit. Explore and savor the benefits.

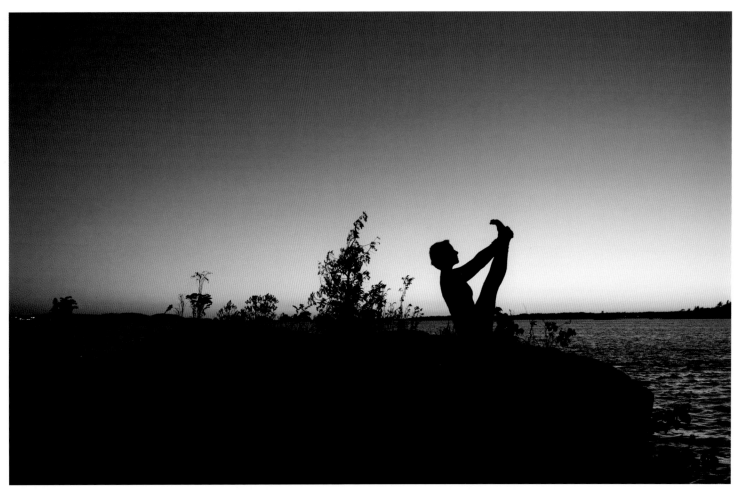

Urdhva Mukha Paschimottanasana I • Upward Facing Intense Stretch to the West Pose

SPIRITUALITY

"I want to give you the depth and the strength which is yours . . . the original you."
YOGI BHAJAN

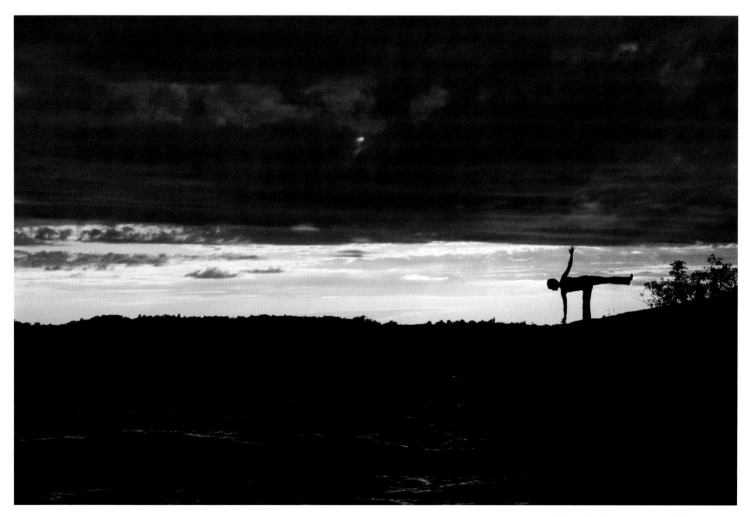

Ardha Chandrasana I • Half Moon Pose

GLOSSARY

Abraham Lincoln – 16th President of the United States known for abolishing slavery

Acupuncture – ancient Chinese medicine utilizing sterilized needles at specific points on the body to alleviate physical, mental, and emotional conditions

Adho – Sanskrit term meaning "downward"

Ahimsa – Sanskrit term meaning "to not injure," promoting non-violence toward all living things

Albert Einstein – developed the general theory of relativity, and arguably, the most revered physicist of the 20th century

Anjali mudra – namaste or prayer seal

Anna Thomas – film screenwriter, producer, and author of the best-selling vegetarian cookbook, *The Vegetarian Epicure*

Anthelme Brillat-Savarin – French politician and lawyer who realized fame as an epicure, or partaker in fine wines and foods

Ardha – Sanskrit term meaning "half"

Aromatherapy – alternative medicinal technique that uses essential oils and plant extracts to improve overall wellbeing

Asana – Sanskrit term meaning "posture" or "pose"

Ashram – place that values community and offers spiritual teachings

Ashtanga – Sanskrit term for a style of yoga that offers a standard flow of postures

Ayurveda – originating in India, a science of life that works to balance the body

B.K.S. Iyengar – yoga guru, founder of Iyengar yoga, known for helping to introduce yoga to the Western world

Baddha – Sanskrit term meaning "bound"

The Beatles – Legendary English rock band

Bandha – Sanskrit term referring to an energy lock or seal in the body

Buddhism – non-theistic religion, teachings of which are guides toward awareness and enlightenment

Chakra – energy center in the human body with linked effects on our physical, mental, and spiritual wellbeing

Chandra – Sanskrit term meaning "moon"

Chi – meaning "energy" or "life force" in traditional Chinese culture

Danda – Sanskrit term meaning "staff" or "rod"

David Swenson – leading Western Ashtanga yoga teacher

Deepak Chopra – Indian-American holistic guru and author

Deity – spiritual god or goddess

Dhanura – Sanskrit term meaning "bow"

Dr. Mikao Usui – known as the founder of Reiki

Eka – Sanskrit term meaning "one"

Essential Oils – liquids derived from plants or other organic sources

Federico Fellini – revered Italian film scriptwriter and director

Garam Masala – blend of spices often used in Indian cooking

Siddhartha Gautama – also known as Gautama Buddha or Buddha, sage and founder of Buddhism

Gratitude – thankfulness, appreciation, and a readiness to return kindness

Gautama Buddha – also known as Siddhartha Gautama or Buddha, sage and founder of Buddhism

Guru – Sanskrit term for "master" or "teacher," often of spiritual practices

Gyan mudra – mudra of unified consciousness

Hala – Sanskrit term meaning "plough"

Hasta – Sanskrit term meaning "hand"

Hatha Yoga – focusing on postures (asanas) and breath (prana), it is the most widely practiced yoga in the world

Helen Keller – Leading humanitarian of the 20th century, author and activist who was blind and deaf

Himalayan Salt – mineral-rich rock salt from Pakistan region that may help regulate water levels in the body

Hinduism – traditions-diverse religion, predominant religion of India

His Holiness the XIV Dalai Lama – named Tenzin Gyatso at birth, he is currently the spiritual leader of Tibet

Homeopathy – ancient, natural method for healing

Inner Spirit – divine energy that exists within all of us

Intention – goal or belief that guides our choices and actions and, with attention, may manifest into reality

John F. Kennedy – 35th President of the United States, assassinated in 1963

Joseph Campbell – Writer and American mythologist

Julia Child – American chef and author known for her bestselling cookbook, *Mastering the Art of French Cooking*

Kapota – Sanskrit term meaning "pigeon"

Karma – philosophy concerning how our actions in the present will have impacts on our futures

Lao Tzu – Chinese philosopher and poet

Mahatma Gandhi – peaceful leader and teacher as well as father of the Indian independence movement

Mantra – repeated word or chant used to help achieve energy balance or concentration

Margaret Mead – celebrated American cultural anthropologist

Marsha Norman – American playwright, screenwriter, and novelist

Meditation – state of deep peace and quiet that leads us to a better sense of awareness or higher spiritual consciousness

Mindfulness – state of being presently aware without judgment

Modification – in this book, it means altering recipes by using more or less of listed ingredients to achieve a finished recipe that fits your needs

Mudra – Sanskrit term referring to a hand position that creates an energy force or seal in the body

Mukha – Sanskrit term meaning "mouth" or "face"

Namaste – Sanskrit greeting that essentially translates to "I bow to you"

Naturopathic Therapy – holistic healing method that often utilizes supplements to aid inherent self-healing functions

Neem Karoli Baba – Hindu guru of the 20th century

Om – sacred mantra chanted to open the "ajna" chakra or "third eye"

Oprah Winfrey – American media mogul, spiritual teacher, and philanthropist

Pada – Sanskrit term meaning "foot" or "leg"

Padma – Sanskrit term meaning "lotus"

Paramahansa Yogananda – Indian yogi and guru who is known for introducing the teachings of meditation and Kriya Yoga to Westerners

Parivrtta – Sanskrit term meaning "revolved" or "turned around"

Parsva – Sanskrit term meaning "side" or "lateral"

Paschima – Sanskrit term meaning "the West"

Patanjali – Yoga philosopher and sage who created the Yoga Sutras

Prana – Sanskrit term meaning "life force" or "breath"

Pranayama – Sanskrit term meaning "extension of the life force" or "breath control"

Prasarita – Sanskrit term meaning "stretched out" or "spread out"

Raja – Sanskrit term meaning "lord" or "king"

Ralph Waldo Emerson – Poet and leader of transcendentalist movement

Raw Foodism (Rawism) – practice of only eating foods that are uncooked or cooked under 115°F, unprocessed foods and often organic

Reflexology – practice of healing massage that focuses on points on the hands and feet

Reiki – healing technique that focuses on channeling energy to achieve physical, mental, or spiritual health

Rice Noodles – noodles made from rice that are often used in Asian cooking

Rick Bass – American author and environmental activist

River Yoga – yoga and wellness center located in the Thousand Islands, New York

Sai Baba – Indian spiritual leader

Salamba – Sanskrit term meaning "supported"

Sanskrit – ancient language of India

Sava – Sanskrit term meaning "corpse"

Sensibility – ability to respond to and appreciate situations and other people

Setu Bandha – Sanskrit term meaning "bridge construction"

Sharon Gannon – celebrated American yoga teacher, spiritual leader, and co-founder of Jivamukti yoga

Shiva – popular Hindu deity known as the "destroyer of illusion"

Shiva Linga mudra – energy charging mudra

Shiva Rea – activist and creator of Prana Flow yoga

Sirsa – Sanskrit term meaning "head"

So Hum – yogic chant meaning "I am that, that I am"

Spiritual Consciousness – awareness of a universal energy, which is inclusive of our inner spirit, and what is truly real

Sri K. Pattabhi Jois – spiritual and yoga guru whose teachings helped to create Ashtanga yoga

Sri Ramakrishna – Indian innovator of religious thought

Srimad Bhagavatam – Puranic text of Hinduism

Steve Jobs – American entrepreneur and former CEO of Apple Inc.

Swami – Sanskrit term for a Hindu male spiritual teacher

Swami Kripalu – spiritual and yoga guru whose teachings helped to create Kripalu yoga

Swami Sivananda – Hindu spiritual teacher whose teachings helped to create Sivananda yoga

Swami Vivekananda – influential spiritual leader and Hindu monk

Tada – Sanskrit term meaning "mountain"

Tahini – paste made from ground sesame seeds

Tamari – soy sauce–like liquid that contains mostly soybeans and a little wheat

Tempeh – protein-rich product made from fermented soybeans

Temple of Kriya Yoga – center based in Chicago, Illinois, offering spiritual services

Thich Nhat Hanh – revered Vietnamese Zen Buddhist monk

Thomas Edison – American inventor

Thomas Keller – celebrated American chef and restaurateur

Thousand (1000) Islands – 1,864 U.S. and Canadian islands in the Saint Lawrence River

Tofu – soybean curd

Ujjayi – Sanskrit term meaning "sounding breath"

Upanishads – collection of Vedic texts

Urdhva – Sanskrit term meaning "raised" or "upward"

Ustra – Sanskrit term meaning "camel"

Ut – Sanskrit term meaning "intense"

Uttarabodhi mudra – mudra of enlightenment

Utthita – Sanskrit term meaning "extended"

Variation – in this book, it means altering recipes by substituting listed ingredients to achieve a finished recipe that fits your needs

Vasistha – name of a legendary sage

Veganism – lifestyle in which one abstains from the consumption of animal products

Vegetarian – lifestyle in which one abstains from the consumption of animal meat

Viparita – Sanskrit term meaning "inversion" or "reversed"

Virahadra – name of a great warrior

Vritti – Sanskrit term for modifications of the mind or whirl-pool

Vrksa – Sanskrit term meaning "tree"

W. Hodding Carter – American journalist

Whole Health – mental, physical, emotional, and spiritual wellbeing

William Henry Channing – American Unitarian clergyman, philosopher, and writer

Yin – According to Chinese philosophy, female principle of the universe, combining with "yang" to create all that comes to be

Yoga – meaning "union," a moving meditation of postures (asanas) and breath (prana)

Yogi – practitioner of the physical and spiritual philosophies of yoga

Yogi Bhajan – spiritual leader who introduced Kundalini yoga to the U.S.

YogiBites – in this book, lessons and teachings that help to unveil principals of yoga, consciousness, and kindness

Zen Master Nan-In – Japanese *master* during the Meiji era (1868–1912)

Zen Proverb – short aphorism that originated from the Japanese school of Mahayana Buddhism, typically emphasizing the value of meditation and intuition

RECIPE INDEX

SUBJECT INDEX

ACKNOWLEDGMENTS

We give very special thanks to our amazing families. Thank you for making us laugh, tasting our finished (and trial) recipes, helping us to clean the kitchen, sharing your ideas, helping to create space for us to write and create this book, and your overall support.

To Blake Price-Kellogg and Jonathan Taylor, thank you for taking brilliant photographs and providing artistic input that helped to elevate the look and feel of this book. Blake, thank you also for sharing your inspirational, back-bending yoga practice and time dedicated to our yoga photo outings.

Thank you to Alex Hess with Skyhorse Publishing for your ongoing support and for helping us to share our story.

We sincerely thank friend and photo editor, Susan Phear. We are grateful for your poignant advice about creating a cohesive story.

Nancy Aubertine and Dory Sheldon, thank you for dedication to editing our book in its early stages as well as your support and friendships.

Thousand Islands, New York, and St. Lawrence River, thank you for providing an extraordinary setting for us to create the visual story of this book. The Native Americans called this area "Manatoana" or the "Garden of the Great Spirit." We, and many others, are very fortunate to continue to honor the Thousand Islands as our spiritual garden and home.

Thank you to Minna Anthony Common Nature Center, Rock Island Lighthouse, the Thousand Islands Land Trust and our friends along The River for providing us with gorgeous locations to take photos.

River Yoga Community, thank you for inspiring this book. We are humbled by and grateful for the outpouring of support from our Yoga Community friends and family.

To our mats . . . Thank you for the lessons.

"May we all be blessed, blessed, blessed, so we may be a blessing unto others."
GOSWAMI KRIYANANDA